The Joint Surgery Guide

*What's Normal, What's Not,
and What Really Matters
After Joint Replacement*

DANIEL BROOKS

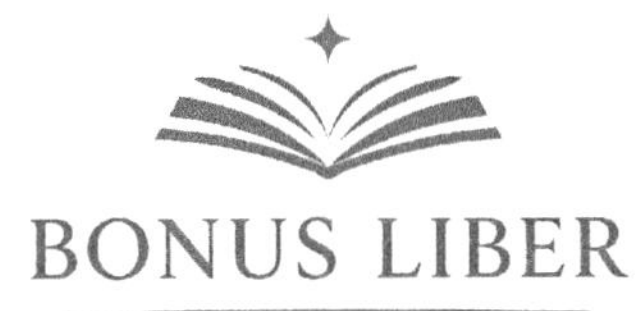

ISBN: 978-1-961963-95-5

Published by Bonus Liber
bonusliber@yourbookshelf.top

Contents

Introduction

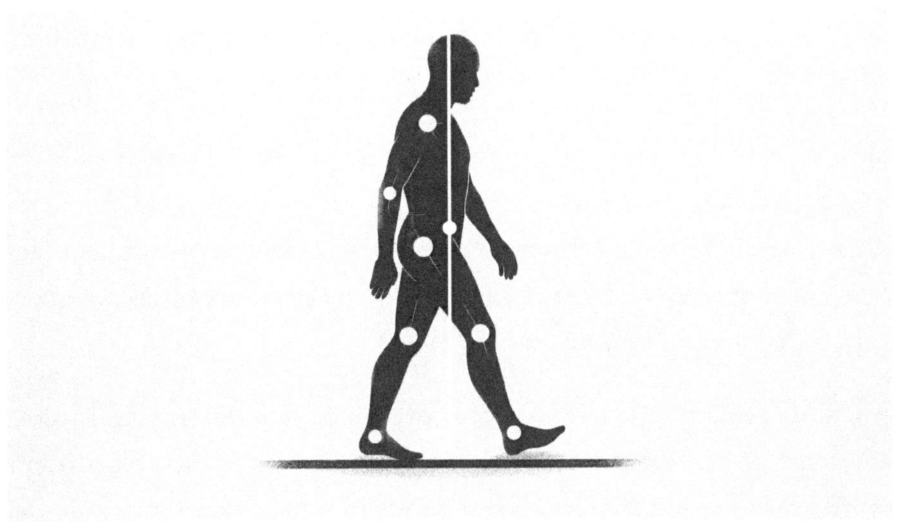

I f you're holding this book, joint pain has likely stopped being something you manage occasionally.
It has started shaping daily choices—how long you stay out, how much
you do, how carefully you plan what used to be simple.

Maybe surgery has already been mentioned. Maybe it hasn't.
Either way, the idea no longer feels distant, and you're probably looking
for clear answers rather than reassurance that doesn't quite match your
experience.

The questions tend to repeat themselves:
What is normal at this point?

What should be improving by now?
And how do you know when something actually needs attention?

Most people reach this stage feeling tired rather than dramatic.
Tired of adjusting plans.
Tired of weighing every activity against how it might feel later.
Tired of hearing that everything "looks fine" while daily life keeps getting harder.

When joint surgery enters the picture, it often brings more uncertainty than relief.

Most information about joint replacement focuses on the procedure itself. This book focuses on what comes before and after—the part patients actually live through. It was written for the moments when appointments are over, advice is brief, and you're left trying to make sense of pain, progress, setbacks, and doubt on your own.

You won't find promises of a perfect recovery here. You also won't find medical jargon or motivational talk. What you will find is a realistic explanation of how recovery usually feels, how it tends to unfold over time, and how to tell the difference between expected discomfort and signals that deserve attention.

This guide is meant for people preparing for or recovering from knee, hip, shoulder, or other major joint replacement surgery. While each joint has its own specifics, many recovery challenges are shared: uneven progress, lingering pain, fatigue, and uncertainty about whether you're doing too much or too little.

The chapters follow the timeline patients describe in real life, not an idealized one. From the moment surgery becomes part of the conversation, through the early days after the procedure, and into the longer phase of recovery that rarely moves in a straight line. Throughout the book, the focus stays on what actually matters: understanding your body, setting realistic expectations, and gradually rebuilding confidence.

This book does not replace medical care. It is meant to support it—by helping you make sense of what you're experiencing and by reducing the constant second-guessing that often comes with recovery.

If you're looking for clarity without false promises, guidance without pressure, and a steadier way to understand what lies ahead, you're in the right place.

BEFORE SURGERY: MAKING SENSE OF THE DECISION

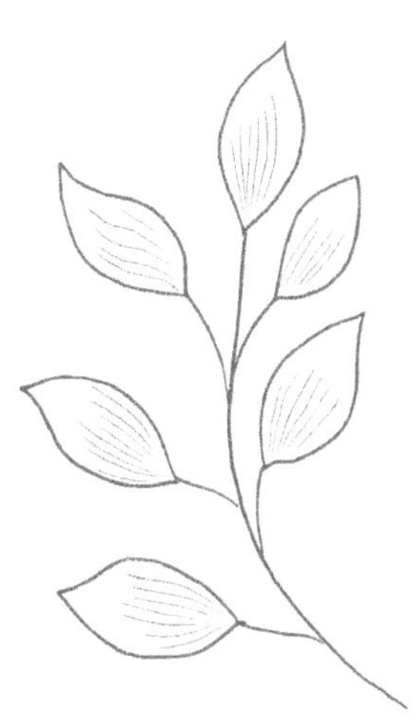

When Surgery Becomes Part of the Conversation

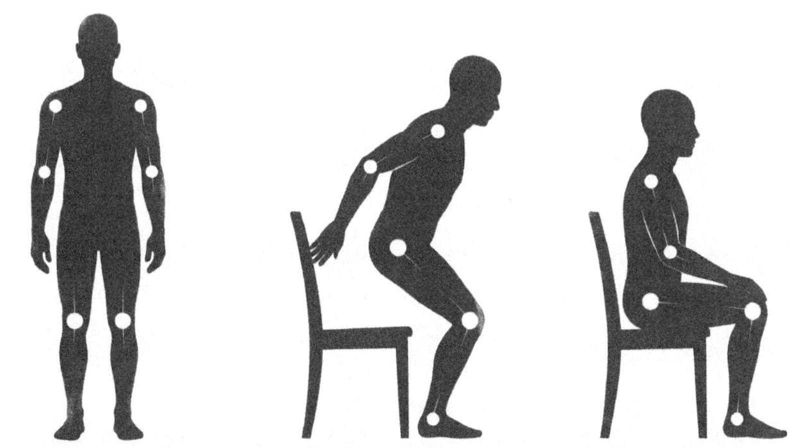

For most people, joint replacement doesn't begin with a decision. It begins with a shift.

At first, pain usually shows up for a reason. A long walk. A day on your feet. A wrong step. You rest, and it settles. You learn which movements to avoid and which positions bring relief. It feels manageable, even if it's frustrating.

Over time, many people notice that pattern changing. Pain doesn't fully leave anymore. It becomes a background presence. Some days it's louder, some days quieter, but it's always there. You don't wait for pain to arrive. You wake up already aware of it.

This is often when daily life starts to narrow. Plans are shaped around what the joint might tolerate. Errands are spaced out. Social events come with an exit plan. Even better days carry caution, because you've learned what often follows.

What surprises many people is how quietly this change happens. There may not be a single injury or clear turning point. Instead, recovery from activity takes longer, and the joint asks for attention more often. Tissues that once settled quickly now stay irritated longer, so small stresses add up instead of clearing overnight.

At some point, a comment is made. A doctor mentions surgery as an option. Or someone asks why you haven't "just had it fixed." That moment often stands out, even though the shift began long before.

Hearing surgery mentioned doesn't mean you're ready. For many people, it creates distance rather than clarity. The idea feels heavy. You may tell yourself it's not that bad, that others have it worse, that you can still manage.

When Management Becomes the Work

Many patients describe this stage as mentally tiring. Not because pain is severe every minute, but because it requires constant calculation. How far is too far. How much is too much. Whether today's soreness means you misjudged something.

Living with a joint that no longer cooperates often means negotiating with your body throughout the day. You test a movement. You wait for feedback. You pull back if it protests. That ongoing back-and-forth takes effort, even when pain levels aren't extreme.

This mental load grows because the joint no longer adapts the way it once did. Muscles around it stay more guarded, and small adjustments stop paying off as reliably. You still compensate, but each adjustment costs more attention and energy than before.

The joint begins to set the pace of your day. You plan around it without fully noticing. You park closer. You avoid certain routes. You sit sooner than you used to. None of these choices feel dramatic, but together they reshape how you move through ordinary life.

What makes this stage difficult is inconsistency. Some days feel almost normal. Others feel heavier for no clear reason. You may loosen up in the morning, then tighten again by evening. That unpredictability keeps you alert, always adjusting.

It's common to minimize this phase, especially if pain isn't constant or severe. You tell yourself you're managing—and you are. The difference is that managing now takes more energy than it returns.

When surgery enters the picture, it often does so because this effort has become exhausting. Management hasn't failed suddenly. Its cost has increased.

Why the Idea of Surgery Feels Heavy

Even when surgery makes sense on paper, it rarely feels neutral. For many people, the idea arrives with a sense of loss that's hard to define.

Part of it is straightforward. Surgery means acknowledging that something hasn't resolved on its own. That time, effort, and patience haven't led where you hoped. For people who value independence, that realization can weigh more than the pain itself.

But the weight isn't only about symptoms.

Surgery introduces an imbalance that's easy to feel and hard to ignore. The costs come first: downtime, dependence, uncertainty. The potential benefits exist later and aren't guaranteed. When effort and risk arrive before relief, hesitation makes sense.

Many people try to counter this by focusing on outcomes. Better movement. Less pain. More freedom. Those possibilities matter, but they don't erase the fact that something must be given up before anything is gained.

There's also the challenge of timing. Even when the body feels ready, life may not be. Work, family responsibilities, and practical constraints all shape how the idea is received. Delay doesn't mean denial; it often reflects the reality of fitting surgery into a life that still has to function.

Because of this, the idea of surgery often feels heavier than expected. Not because it's wrong, but because it asks for trust before it offers proof.

That weight doesn't need to be resolved here. Recognizing it is enough. When the feeling is named, it becomes easier to hold without letting it dominate the decision.

How the Decision Takes Shape Over Time

Very few people wake up certain about surgery. More often, the decision takes shape slowly, in pieces.

You think about it, then set it aside. A good week makes it feel unnecessary. A bad day brings it back. The same questions replay, without a clear answer.

This back-and-forth is common. Surgery isn't chosen in a single moment of clarity. It's weighed over time, alongside daily experience. Each flare, each limitation, each adjustment adds context, even if it doesn't feel decisive when it happens.

Many people expect a clear threshold—*when it gets bad enough, I'll know.* In reality, that line is rarely sharp. Pain shifts. Function changes unevenly. Some parts of life stay manageable while others quietly narrow.

What often moves the decision forward isn't a sudden worsening, but accumulation. The growing effort required to keep things running. The sense that managing now takes more energy than it gives back. Life starts organizing itself around a problem that isn't improving.

There's also the time it takes to accept the idea itself. Surgery challenges how people see themselves: capable, independent, reliable. Adjusting that self-image doesn't happen quickly.

Practical factors matter too. Family input. Work schedules. Insurance. Care responsibilities. Even when the body feels ready, timing may not be. That delay doesn't cancel the decision; it reflects real constraints.

Some people notice progress when the question shifts. Not *Will this fix everything?* but *Is this how I want to keep living?* The change is subtle, but it reframes the choice.

By the time surgery becomes a concrete plan, many people realize the decision has been forming for a while. They simply needed time to recognize it.

That time is part of the process, not a detour.

Naming the Moment Without Forcing the Answer

When surgery enters the conversation, it isn't a verdict. It's a signal that the strategies that once worked no longer cover the full cost.

This chapter isn't about pushing you toward a choice. It's about naming the point where managing stops being neutral and starts demanding more than it gives back. Understanding how you reached this place helps separate effort from failure, and attention from weakness.

For many people, that understanding brings a small sense of relief. Not because the answer is suddenly clear, but because the experience finally has a shape. What felt vague and draining becomes easier to recognize and talk about.

Nothing needs to be decided here. This is simply the moment where the question appears, often quietly, and begins to stay.

2

What Joint Replacement Can — and Cannot — Do

Most people imagine improvement after joint replacement as a clean exchange. Pain out, function in. The joint is replaced, healing happens, and daily life resumes with fewer limits. That picture isn't wrong, but it's incomplete.

Improvement usually arrives in pieces. One change shows up here, another there, often without a clear turning point. You might notice you can stand a little longer before sitting, or that sleep feels slightly less broken. Pain may still be present, but it behaves differently. It takes up less space. It stops running every decision.

This matters because many people expect improvement to announce itself clearly. They wait for a moment when things are obviously better. When that moment doesn't arrive, it's easy to assume nothing is changing. In reality, change is often quiet and uneven.

Pain relief and functional improvement do not always move together. You may move more easily while still feeling sore or stiff. You may tolerate activity better even though discomfort hasn't settled yet. If progress has always been judged by pain alone, this disconnect can feel confusing.

What often shifts first is how predictable the joint feels. Daily activities involve fewer surprises. There's less bracing before movement. Limits still exist, but they stop dominating attention. Pain begins to loosen its hold before it fully steps back.

These early changes are easy to miss because they don't feel dramatic. But they matter. They signal that the joint is starting to fit into daily life instead of interrupting it. That is often the first real sign that improvement is underway.

The Limits That Come With the Change

Joint replacement can do a lot, but it does not return the body to an earlier version of itself. That distinction is not always clear before surgery, even when expectations are discussed. Most people hear what the procedure is meant to fix. Fewer hear what may remain.

The joint surface is new. The rest of the system is not. Muscles, tendons, nerves, balance, and long-standing movement habits have often adapted to pain over years. Those adaptations do not reset just because the joint has been replaced.

This explains why some sensations feel unfamiliar afterward. Deep joint pain may ease, while nearby areas feel irritated or tight. Muscles that were underused can fatigue quickly. Others that carried extra load before surgery may stay guarded. None of this means the joint is failing. It reflects how the surrounding tissues are adjusting to a different mechanical environment.

A replaced joint also sends different signals. Pressure, stiffness, or a vague sense of resistance may not register as pain, but they can still feel noticeable. Some people have small numb areas near the incision. These sensations often fade, but not always completely. The goal of surgery is improvement, not erasing every signal from the area.

Endurance is another common surprise. Strength may return sooner than stamina. An activity may feel manageable once, but repeating it several times in a day can be harder. Tissues that have been stressed, protected, or altered for a long time tend to tire more easily at first.

When these limits aren't explained, they're easy to misread. Lingering discomfort can feel like damage. Fatigue can feel like regression. Most of the time, they reflect adjustment rather than a problem.

Joint replacement is very effective at reducing certain pain and improving basic function. It is less effective at removing every trace of how the body learned to cope before surgery. Understanding that difference early often makes the experience steadier. When sensations make sense, they carry less weight.

Pain Relief and Function Don't Move Together

One of the most common surprises after joint replacement is how loosely pain relief and function are connected. Many people expect pain to improve first and movement to follow. Often, the opposite happens.

Function can improve while pain is still present. You may walk farther, stand longer, or move more smoothly even though soreness or stiffness lingers. If pain has always been the main signal guiding your choices, this can feel contradictory.

Before surgery, pain usually stops movement directly. After surgery, discomfort is more often reactive. It shows up later, after activity, rather than blocking you right away. That shift can make it harder to judge what the joint can handle.

Pain after surgery is influenced by more than the joint itself. Healing tissue, swelling, and a sensitive nervous system all affect how things feel. Because of this, pain is not always a clear indicator of structural stress or progress.

Two people can report the same level of pain and have very different functional ability. That's why improvement is often easier to see in what you can do than in how things feel moment to moment.

It's also common for pain to vary even when activity stays similar. A good morning doesn't guarantee an easy evening. These swings are part of how the body adapts to change.

Understanding that pain relief and function follow different paths helps set more realistic expectations. It allows gains to register even when discomfort hasn't fully settled. For many people, function begins to pull ahead first. Pain tends to follow later.

A Different Kind of Normal

Before surgery, many people picture recovery as a return to how the joint felt years ago. The same ease. The same range. The sense that the joint disappears completely. For some, parts of that return. For most, what develops is something slightly different.

The joint usually becomes quieter, but not invisible. It stops dominating attention, yet it still makes itself known at times. Certain movements feel different. Long days leave a trace that wasn't there before. These changes can feel disappointing if the goal was to forget the joint entirely.

What often improves most is predictability. Before surgery, pain interrupts without warning. After things settle, the joint behaves more consistently. You learn what it tolerates well and what needs spacing. That consistency makes daily planning easier, even if the joint is not perfect.

Comfort also tends to vary by situation. Many people find walking easier than standing still, or movement easier than rest. These patterns aren't intuitive, but they are common and often become part of the baseline.

Over time, awareness shifts. Early on, every sensation feels important. Later, many fade into the background. They don't disappear, but they stop demanding constant interpretation. That change alone reduces mental load.

Noticing the joint occasionally does not mean recovery is incomplete. Many well-functioning joints still send signals. The difference is that those signals no longer control behavior.

This version of normal is not about erasing limits. It is about having clearer, more manageable ones. For most people, that trade turns out to be easier to live with than the unpredictability that came before.

Expectations That Quietly Complicate Things

Some expectations sound reasonable but add strain over time. They turn normal variation into doubt and ordinary limits into frustration.

One of the most common is the idea that improvement should be steady. When progress slows or briefly reverses, it's easy to assume something is wrong. In reality, change often happens in uneven steps, especially as activity increases.

Timing expectations create similar trouble. Many people carry mental deadlines for when pain should be gone or movement should feel normal. These timelines are often borrowed from someone else's experience or simplified explanations. Bodies don't follow calendars very well.

There is also the belief that effort controls outcome in a direct way. That if everything is done "right," recovery will respond predictably. Effort matters, but healing still moves at its own pace. Pushing harder does not always speed improvement, and pulling back does not automatically slow it.

Another expectation is that the joint will give clear signals. Pain means stop. No pain means go. After surgery, feedback is less clean. Swelling, fatigue, and sensitivity blur the message. Misreading those signals at times is common and does not mean failure.

Comparison adds pressure. Hearing about someone else's fast progress can make your own feel inadequate. Those comparisons usually miss differences in history, daily demands, or support.

Letting go of these expectations is not about lowering standards. It's about choosing ones that fit how recovery actually works. When expectations soften, progress is easier to recognize without measuring it against an imagined version of how it should look.

Clarity Before the Decision

Deciding on joint replacement is rarely about a single bad day. It's usually about a long stretch of adjustment. Plans change. Pain gets managed quietly. Daily life becomes smaller in ways that aren't always visible to others.

Clarity matters because surgery is not a rescue from one problem. It's a trade. One set of limits is exchanged for another, usually more workable, set. When that trade is understood, the decision tends to feel steadier.

Many people wait for certainty. They want assurance that the outcome will justify the effort. That assurance doesn't exist. What helps more is knowing what the procedure reliably improves and what it does not. Reducing constant joint pain and improving basic function are realistic goals. Returning to an untouched body is not.

Clarity also means being honest about what you hope to regain. For some, it's walking without planning every step. For others, it's sleeping with fewer interruptions or managing daily tasks with less drain. These goals are practical, and they usually line up with what joint replacement can offer.

This decision doesn't require optimism. It requires realism. When surgery is understood as a process rather than a fix, setbacks feel less surprising and progress invites less second-guessing.

Pain often narrows life gradually. Surgery is usually considered when that narrowing becomes too costly to maintain. Not dramatic. Just no longer workable.

Clarity before the decision doesn't remove uncertainty. It changes how you relate to it. Instead of asking whether surgery will be perfect, the question becomes whether continuing as you are still makes sense. For many people, that shift brings a quiet sense of resolve rather than excitement.

3

Preparing Your Body (Without Doing Too Much)

When surgery is scheduled, many people naturally shift into preparation mode. If something big is coming, it makes sense to want to feel ready. Strength often becomes the focus. Stronger muscles sound like they should lead to an easier recovery, and that idea is reinforced by well-meaning advice.

In reality, preparing the body before surgery is rarely that straightforward. Most people arrive at this point already living with pain that has shaped how they move. One side may be weaker, another tighter. Certain muscles have been working overtime to protect a joint that no longer moves well. Over time, these compensations stop feeling temporary and start to feel normal.

When preparation is framed only as "getting stronger," people often push straight into those existing patterns. They do more of what the body already uses to cope. Instead of balancing things out, this can increase strain on irritated tissue, add swelling, and create fatigue in the weeks before surgery.

There is often an emotional layer underneath this effort. Preparation can quietly turn into proof that you are doing everything right, that you are not giving in, that you will be the one who recovers quickly. None of that is intentional, but it adds pressure.

This is usually where preparation stops helping.

Before surgery, strength is not about reaching a peak. It is about arriving in a state the body can tolerate. Calm, familiar, and not worn down. Surgeons and therapists often see that people who exhaust themselves trying to prepare perfectly struggle more afterward. Not because effort is wrong, but because recovery asks for reserves, not output.

Another common misunderstanding is assuming that pain during preparation signals progress. Before surgery, pain carries different information. A joint that is already damaged does not adapt the way a healthy joint does. Pushing through pain in this phase usually teaches the body to guard more, not move better. That guarding tends to show up later as stiffness or hesitation in early recovery.

Preparation that truly helps often looks quieter than expected. It focuses on keeping movement familiar rather than forcing change. It respects fatigue instead of challenging it. It values consistency over intensity.

This does not mean doing nothing. It means understanding what the body can actually use. In the weeks before surgery, your system is already under stress. Pain affects sleep. Appointments and decisions pile up. Uncertainty is constant. Adding extra physical strain on top of that can tip the balance in subtle ways that only show up later.

Many people expect confidence to come from having trained hard. More often, it comes from knowing your limits and staying within them. If preparation leaves you more tired than usual, more sore day after day, or constantly second-guessing whether you are doing enough, that is useful information. It does not mean you have failed. It means your body is already working hard.

Some people find relief when they reframe preparation as preservation. Keeping movement within comfortable ranges. Maintaining routines that do not spike pain. Letting the body stay familiar with daily tasks instead of chasing improvement. Surgery is not a test of effort. It is a transition.

Arriving steady matters more than arriving strong. Before surgery, giving the body space is part of preparation too.

When Preparation Starts to Backfire

Most people don't notice when preparation quietly crosses a line. There is rarely a clear moment where it becomes obvious. Instead, small changes begin to accumulate.

Pain that used to settle now lingers. Swelling appears more easily. Sleep feels lighter or more broken. Thoughts about the joint take up more space, with constant checking and quiet worry about whether enough is being done. Preparation starts to feel heavier than it should.

Before surgery, the joint is still damaged. It does not respond to overload by getting stronger. Instead, it becomes more protective. Muscles tighten, movement narrows, and the body braces. That bracing can feel like strength, but underneath it is working harder just to maintain basic function.

This is often where reasonable effort turns into strain. Each activity may feel manageable on its own, but the body does not fully return to baseline between efforts. Irritation builds gradually. Fatigue becomes constant rather than occasional.

Another sign preparation is no longer helping is when rest begins to feel unproductive. Some people feel uneasy on days they do less, as if they are losing ground. Better days start to feel fragile, and harder days linger longer than before.

The early signals are usually subtle. Swelling that takes longer to calm. Heaviness that carries into the next day. Sleep that worsens even as effort increases. None of these are alarming on their own, but together they matter.

As surgery approaches, overall stress naturally rises. Appointments, logistics, and uncertainty add load. If physical preparation keeps escalating at the same time, the system does not get a break. That matters because early recovery depends on reserve. A body that arrives already worn down has less room to adapt.

Noticing this does not mean stopping everything. It often means allowing soreness to fully settle and letting easier days stay easy. Preparation backfires most often when a reasonable approach is carried on for too long without adjustment.

Catching that early can change how the next phase feels.

The Fine Line Between Helpful and Harmful Effort

Preparation rarely becomes unhelpful because it is extreme. More often, it slips past a narrow line without being noticed. Before surgery, the body is already adapting around a problem joint. Muscles are compensating. Movements are adjusted automatically. When effort increases, those patterns tend to deepen rather than correct. The body chooses protection over efficiency.

Helpful effort supports what you already do reasonably well. Harmful effort tries to force change in a system that does not have the capacity to change right now. That line is not defined by numbers. It shows up in response. How you feel later that day. How you feel the next morning. How quickly things settle back to your usual level.

One way people cross this line is by stacking demands. Each activity feels manageable on its own, so they are combined. A walk, some focused movement, errands, all in the same day. Together, they exceed what the joint can absorb. The reaction is often delayed, showing up as stiffness or swelling that lingers.

Another common pattern is pushing hardest on better days. When pain is quieter, it feels like an opportunity to catch up. The problem is that good days are often fragile. Loading them heavily tends to trigger harder days that follow. Helpful effort leaves room for fluctuation. Harmful effort tries to smooth it out.

There is usually a mental shift as well. Preparation starts to feel urgent. Missing a day creates anxiety. Rest feels like falling behind. These reactions are not a sign of poor motivation. They are signs that the process has become heavier than it needs to be.

In clinical settings, this is often where people ask, "Am I doing enough?" A more useful question is whether the body is recovering between efforts. Before surgery, recovery looks like returning to baseline by the next day. It looks like swelling that comes and goes, not swelling that accumulates. It looks like sleep that is disrupted by pain, but not steadily worse because of activity.

Helpful effort supports those patterns. Harmful effort erodes them gradually. Narrowing the focus during this phase often helps. Fewer demands, repeated consistently, are usually better tolerated than many demands done occasionally. This reduces both physical strain and mental load.

What matters most is not how hard you are trying. It is whether your body can settle afterward. That ability to reset is one of the clearest signs that preparation is still serving you rather than draining you.

Letting the Body Arrive, Not Peak

As surgery gets closer, many people feel the urge to make one last push. One more week of effort. One more attempt to feel fully ready. There is comfort in believing that a bit more work will improve the outcome.

The body does not benefit from arriving at surgery at its limit. This phase is better thought of as allowing things to settle. Not in a technical way, but in how you treat your energy and your joint. The aim is not to build momentum. It is to reduce noise.

When strain eases, irritation often settles with it. Swelling becomes less reactive. Muscles soften instead of bracing. Movement feels more predictable. None of this looks impressive, but it creates a steadier starting point.

This matters because surgery interrupts everything. The nervous system has to recalibrate. Basic movement has to be relearned. A body that is not already overloaded adapts more easily, even if nothing about preparation looked remarkable.

Some people worry that easing off means losing progress. In reality, very little meaningful conditioning is lost close to surgery. What tends to be lost when pushing continues is tolerance. Sensitivity increases. Fatigue accumulates. Confidence quietly erodes.

Letting the body arrive means allowing days that feel uneventful. Movement that does not challenge. Rest that does not need to be earned. It means trusting that maintaining function is enough.

This can be uncomfortable for people who measure readiness by output. Steps taken. Time spent moving. Surgery asks for a different kind of readiness, one that is harder to quantify.

Arrival is about familiarity. Your body knows how to get through the day. It recognizes what feels safe. It is not constantly reacting.

In the final stretch, many people notice that when effort softens, pain does not vanish, but it becomes less sharp. Sleep steadies slightly. The joint feels less reactive. These are small shifts, but they matter.

You do not need to peak for surgery. You need to show up with something left to work with.

A Calmer Kind of Readiness

When people picture being "ready" for surgery, they often imagine confidence built on action. Things completed. Effort applied. A sense that everything possible has been done.

Many patients later describe a different kind of readiness as more helpful. Not confidence from doing more, but calm from stability. This shows up quietly. You have a sense of what your joint tolerates and you tend to stay within that range. Fluctuations feel familiar rather than alarming. Good days are not chased, and harder days are not treated as failures.

This kind of readiness does not remove anxiety. Surgery is still surgery. What it reduces is the constant background tension that comes from monitoring yourself and second-guessing every choice. The body is not being asked to perform. It is being allowed to hold steady.

When preparation quiets down, many people notice that decisions feel easier. There is less reactivity, less pressure to adjust or add something. That mental space becomes important later, especially in the early weeks after surgery when sensations, instructions, and emotions can feel like a lot at once.

A calmer readiness also changes the relationship with discomfort. Pain is still present, but it is no longer treated as a problem to fix or push through. It is something you already understand. That familiarity tends to reduce guarding, which helps movement feel less threatening.

This approach is sometimes mistaken for lowering standards. It is not. It is matching effort to what the body can actually use. Recovery responds to steadiness, not intensity.

Before surgery, readiness often comes from doing a little less, not more. Letting preparation fit into life rather than take it over. Allowing quiet days to be enough.

Being ready does not always feel active. Sometimes it feels settled.

4

Preparing Your Mind for Recovery

Most preparation before surgery focuses on logistics and the body. Appointments. Tests. Exercises. What to bring. What to stop eating. What to arrange at home. That part is visible and concrete.

Much less attention is given to what happens internally once the date is fixed. For many people, that's when things feel subtly unsettled. Not dramatic. Just slightly off. Thoughts circle more easily. Sleep may feel lighter. Small decisions take more effort. Even when nothing specific is wrong, there can be a sense of waiting without knowing for what.

This often surprises people because it doesn't look like fear in the usual sense. You may feel calm on the surface. You may even feel relieved to have a plan. And yet, something keeps running quietly in the background.

What's happening is not emotional weakness or doubt about the decision. It's the nervous system adjusting to a known disruption. Once surgery is scheduled, the brain shifts from problem-solving to anticipation. It starts monitoring for change, even before anything has changed yet.

Surgery also represents a pause in normal control. Your body will be acted on. Your schedule will narrow. Your independence will temporarily shrink.

Even when these things are expected and accepted, the system still registers them as a change in status.

Most people don't talk about this phase because it feels vague and hard to justify. There's no single symptom to point to. No clear problem to solve. But it's common, and it's real.

This chapter focuses on that quieter side of preparation. Not because it needs fixing, but because understanding it usually reduces confusion. When reactions have an explanation, they tend to feel less heavy.

Sometimes, simply knowing what is happening is enough to steady it.

Fear That Doesn't Match the Facts

Once surgery is scheduled, fear often shows up in ways people don't expect. Not as panic or dread, but as a low-level unease that doesn't seem proportional to the situation.

You may know the procedure is common. You may trust your surgeon. You may feel clear that surgery is the right step. And still, something feels unsettled.

This can be confusing, and sometimes embarrassing. When nothing specific is wrong, people often tell themselves they're overreacting. Others try to push the feeling aside by focusing harder on details and plans.

But this kind of fear isn't driven by logic. It comes from anticipation. The nervous system is designed to scan ahead for potential threat, especially when something significant is coming that can't be fully predicted or rehearsed.

Surgery concentrates several uncertainties at once. Physical sensation. Loss of routine. Temporary dependence on others. The unknown pace of recovery. Even when each piece makes sense on its own, together they activate vigilance without a clear target.

That's why this fear often has no single focus. It may show up at night, when the day quiets down and there's less distraction. Thoughts loop. Sleep feels lighter. Or it may appear as irritability, restlessness, or a sense of detachment. These are different expressions of the same process.

Another reason this fear feels unsettling is that it fluctuates. One conversation reassures you. Another raises new questions. A good day makes surgery feel unnecessary. A harder day makes it feel urgent. That back-and-forth is tiring, even when nothing has changed.

This pattern doesn't mean you're unsure about your decision. It means your system is reacting to a loss of predictability. For people who rely on planning and adjustment to feel steady, that loss can feel particularly uncomfortable.

Fear before surgery is not always a warning signal. More often, it's the brain trying to prepare for something that cannot be fully mapped in advance.

When this reaction is treated as a problem to eliminate, it often intensifies. When it's understood as part of the transition, it usually softens. Not because it disappears, but because it stops feeling like a sign that something is wrong.

Fear that doesn't seem to make sense is still a real nervous-system response. Recognizing that can take some pressure off at a time when pressure is already high.

Losing Control, Even for a While

One of the quieter strains before surgery is the awareness that control is about to narrow. Not permanently, but enough to be felt.

Even people who feel steady about the procedure often react to this in small ways. You may catch yourself thinking about who will help you at home, how much you'll need to ask for, or what it will feel like to wait for permission to move, shower, or drive. These thoughts don't always come with worry attached. They just keep returning.

Most adults spend years adapting around limitations without naming them. They compensate. They adjust. They stay independent. Surgery interrupts that pattern. For a period of time, your body won't respond in familiar ways, regardless of preparation.

This shift can register as impatience or irritability rather than fear. Some people become more focused on organizing and planning, as if precision could offset uncertainty. When that sense of control slips anyway, tension builds.

Control is closely tied to identity. Being capable. Being reliable. Being the one others lean on. Surgery temporarily reverses that role. You become the one who waits, who follows instructions, who needs assistance. Even when this is expected, it can feel unsettling.

These reactions don't signal low resilience. They reflect adjustment. The nervous system tracks changes in autonomy just as closely as it tracks physical threat.

People respond to this in different ways. Some minimize it by telling themselves it will be brief. Others avoid thinking about dependence at all. Both responses are common. Both can make the early days feel more jarring when intention doesn't translate into action.

Many patients say the hardest moments aren't the procedure itself, but the first days afterward, when effort doesn't lead to immediate results. You want to move, but can't easily. You want to help, but are told to rest. The mismatch between desire and ability is frustrating.

Understanding that this phase is expected helps orient the experience. Control doesn't vanish. It contracts, then gradually returns.

Preparation at this stage isn't about preventing that feeling. It's about knowing why it shows up, so it doesn't feel alarming when it does.

When control narrows, patience matters more than strength. And patience comes less from willpower than from knowing what reactions are typical in this transition.

Why Uncertainty Feels So Draining

Pain is familiar. You feel it, you respond to it, and over time you learn its patterns. Uncertainty works differently. It has no clear edges, and it keeps asking for attention.

As surgery approaches, many people notice that uncertainty is more exhausting than discomfort itself. You don't know exactly how the first days will feel. You don't know how quickly things will improve, or which parts will be harder than expected. Even when you've been given information, there is a gap between knowing something in theory and living it.

That gap takes energy.

When the future is unclear, the brain stays active. It replays conversations. It runs scenarios. It checks and rechecks for signs of readiness. This doesn't feel dramatic, but it uses mental resources steadily throughout the day. By evening, you may feel worn out without having done much at all.

This is why people sometimes feel more fatigued before surgery, even if pain hasn't changed. The body is managing its usual load, while the mind is managing possibility. Together, they increase overall strain.

Uncertainty also removes reference points. With pain, you can compare today to yesterday. With the future, there is nothing solid to measure against. Reassurance fades quickly because the next unknown is always waiting.

Many patients are surprised by the sense of relief that follows surgery, even during early recovery. Not because things are easy, but because uncertainty collapses into reality. You know what hurts. You know what you can and cannot do. The constant guessing stops.

Before surgery, uncertainty is unavoidable. Feeling more tired, distracted, or irritable during this phase doesn't mean you're handling things poorly. It means your system is carrying extra load.

Recognizing that can reduce self-judgment. The fatigue isn't a personal shortcoming. It's a predictable response to prolonged uncertainty.

Information and the Need for Orientation

As surgery approaches, many people feel a strong pull toward information. Not out of curiosity, but out of a need for orientation.

When something important is coming and the outcome can't be fully predicted, the brain looks for structure. Information provides that. It doesn't remove uncertainty, but it gives it edges. It turns a vague threat into something more defined.

This is why broad reassurance often feels unsatisfying. "You'll be fine" offers little to hold onto. Clear, realistic explanation tends to help more. Not because it promises comfort, but because it reduces surprise.

Knowing that pain may increase before it settles. That fatigue is common. That progress rarely moves in a straight line. These details don't make recovery easy, but they make it recognizable.

At the same time, more information isn't always better. Endless searching can keep the nervous system in a state of alert, especially when stories conflict or focus on extremes. Orientation comes from grounded, contextual information, not volume.

Many people notice that the most helpful explanations answer questions they didn't yet know how to ask. What the first night is usually like. What tends to feel hardest. Which worries often show up later rather than right away.

When information reduces guessing, vigilance eases. Sensations feel less alarming. Reactions feel less personal. You stop scanning constantly for signs that something is wrong.

This is one of the roles of this book. Not to prepare you perfectly, but to reduce the sense of walking into the unknown without any reference points.

Information doesn't erase uncertainty. It makes it easier to carry.

Expectations and Mental Load

As surgery gets closer, expectations often tighten without much notice. You picture how recovery should unfold. How quickly you should move. How much better you should feel at each step. Even when you try not to compare, other timelines and stories tend to slip in.

These expectations rarely show up as clear rules. They sit quietly in the background and shape how you interpret what happens. When things line up, they go unnoticed. When they don't, tension builds.

Before surgery, expectations are mostly theoretical. They're formed from partial information, brief conversations, and other people's experiences. Once recovery begins, those expectations meet reality, and reality is rarely consistent.

When expectations are rigid, normal variation can feel like failure. A slower day may feel like a setback. A flare in discomfort can feel like a sign that something is wrong. The mental effort of checking progress against an internal standard adds to overall fatigue.

Allowing expectations to stay flexible reduces that load. Not by lowering hope, but by leaving room for unevenness. Recovery rarely follows a straight line, and the nervous system reacts less strongly when change doesn't feel like a violation of the plan.

This flexibility becomes especially important when progress slows or stalls. Without it, the mind fills gaps with worry. With it, the same pauses feel easier to tolerate.

Before surgery, noticing expectations can be enough. Recognizing that many of them are guesses, not guarantees, helps keep them from becoming a source of pressure.

Expectations don't disappear. They loosen. And when they do, there is more space to adapt to what actually unfolds.

5

Getting Your Home Ready

When people start getting their home ready for surgery, attention often goes straight to equipment. Chairs, tools, and products meant to make recovery easier. Lining these things up can feel reassuring, especially when so much else feels uncertain.

Some preparation does help. But many patients later notice that the items they worried about most played a smaller role than expected. What mattered more was how the space felt to move through when energy was low.

Before surgery, recovery is often imagined as a problem that can be solved by having the right setup. If everything is in place, the first days should go smoothly. That idea offers a sense of control at a time when control already feels limited.

In real life, the first days are shaped less by gear and more by comfort and effort. How far you need to walk. How easily you can sit or lie down. How simple it is to rest without rearranging yourself each time. These details tend to matter more than specialized items.

Many people gather far more than they end up using. At the same time, they're often surprised by how tiring clutter, noise, and extra decisions feel. After surgery, tolerance is lower. The body is already using energy to heal, and the brain tires more quickly when it has to navigate obstacles or choices.

Preparing your home works best when the goal is reducing friction. Fewer obstacles. Fewer decisions. A space that supports rest and easy movement without asking for constant adjustment.

When preparation is framed this way, it often feels lighter. You're not trying to solve every possible problem in advance. You're simply shaping the space so it asks less of you during a demanding phase.

What Actually Gets Used

Once people are home after surgery, priorities tend to shift quickly. What seemed essential beforehand often fades into the background, while a few simple things get used again and again.

What usually matters most is access, not equipment. A clear path to the bathroom. A stable place to sit. A surface within easy reach for water, medication, or a phone. These everyday details shape how manageable the first days feel.

Many patients are surprised by how little tolerance they have for unnecessary movement. Bending, reaching, and navigating around furniture take more effort than expected. Items that are technically helpful lose value if they require extra steps or awkward positioning. The body spends more energy on balance and coordination after surgery, which makes small movements feel bigger than they used to.

Comfort also changes meaning. A chair that looks supportive may feel wrong once swelling and stiffness set in. Beds, couches, and armchairs are often adjusted on the fly. What works on day one may feel different on day three. Being able to make small changes tends to matter more than any single "ideal" setup.

People often ask what they should buy. In practice, it's more useful to notice what you reach for when you're tired and sore. Things you already use and trust tend to feel easiest. Familiarity reduces both physical effort and mental load, especially when concentration is limited.

Many patients later notice that the most-used items were simple ones: a firm pillow, a stable chair, a clear surface, a short walking path. The rest either stayed unused or felt optional.

Preparing with this in mind shifts the focus away from collecting and toward arranging. The goal isn't to add more to the home, but to let what's already there work better for you.

The First Days at Home

The transition from the hospital to home is often more demanding than people expect. In the hospital, movement is guided and help is close. The environment is built around recovery. At home, familiar spaces suddenly require more effort.

The first days tend to feel narrow. Not in a dramatic way, but in how much energy even simple tasks take. Standing up, walking a short distance, getting comfortable again—each step asks for attention. Many people are surprised by how quickly they feel tired, even when pain is controlled. This happens because surgery temporarily lowers stamina and the brain has to work harder to coordinate movement.

This isn't a setback. It's a common response to both surgery and the shift in responsibility that happens once you're home.

At home, you're no longer moving on cue. You decide when to get up, when to rest, and when to try again. That freedom can feel good, but it also adds mental load. You're constantly checking in with your body and deciding whether something is worth the effort.

During this phase, days often feel repetitive. You move, you rest, and you repeat. Progress shows up in small ways: getting back to a chair with less effort, needing fewer adjustments to get comfortable, recovering a little faster after each attempt.

Many people expect pain to be the hardest part. More often, it's coordination. The body feels unfamiliar. Timing is off. Movements that once flowed now happen in steps. This can feel frustrating, especially if you expected to feel more capable right away.

Sleep also tends to be unsettled at first. Rest may come in shorter stretches, and positions often need frequent changes. This is common early on and usually settles gradually rather than all at once.

Emotionally, the first days at home can feel quieter but heavier. There's less distraction and more time to notice sensations. Small worries can feel larger when energy is low.

In this window, the goal isn't productivity or independence. It's stability. Finding a rhythm your body can tolerate so the days feel manageable rather than demanding.

Small adjustments in the home make a difference here. Fewer trips across the room. Less decision-making. More time spent resting without interruption. These choices don't slow recovery. They support it.

Small Changes That Reduce Friction

In the early phase of recovery, effort adds up quickly. What feels minor before surgery can feel heavy afterward. That's why small environmental changes often matter more than people expect.

Friction usually comes from repetition. Walking the same short path many times a day. Standing up and sitting down again and again. Reaching, turning, adjusting. Each action on its own seems insignificant. Together, they shape how tiring the day feels.

Reducing friction doesn't require major rearranging. It starts with noticing where effort clusters and softening those points. Shorter distances help. Clearer walkways reduce the need to watch every step. Stable surfaces make transitions feel steadier when balance and strength are temporarily reduced.

Chairs are a common example. A seat that's slightly too low or too soft can turn every stand-up into a strain. Small adjustments in firmness or height often change how much energy is spent just getting up. The same is true for beds and couches. Minor changes can affect how often you need to reposition yourself.

Bathrooms tend to concentrate effort. Limited space, hard surfaces, and awkward angles demand attention when coordination is off. Simplifying the space—fewer items in the way, clearer placement—can make these moments feel less tense.

Noise and interruptions also add friction. Constant activity, repeated questions, or background sound can be more draining than expected. Many people do better with predictable quiet periods where rest isn't interrupted.

What often helps most is thinking in terms of flow. How you move from one task to the next. Where you pause. Where you recover. When the environment supports that flow, the day feels steadier even if nothing else changes.

These adjustments aren't permanent. They temporarily reshape the space to match a lower energy level. People who reduce friction often describe the early weeks as less exhausting, even when pain levels are similar.

The body still works hard. It just isn't fighting the environment at the same time.

Letting the Space Support You

In the first weeks after surgery, the space around you has more influence than it might seem. When energy is limited, the environment either absorbs effort or demands it.

A supportive space doesn't draw attention to itself. You can move through it without planning every step or negotiating each transition. When things are where you expect them to be, your body spends less energy compensating, and rest feels more complete.

This matters because recovery temporarily lowers tolerance for both physical effort and decision-making. Familiar layouts reduce the mental work of navigating the day, which helps preserve energy for movement and healing. Small choices—clear paths, fewer obstacles, items within easy reach—quiet that background strain.

For some people, adjusting the home brings up an unexpected concern: that these changes mean settling into a smaller version of life. In practice, the opposite is usually true. Temporary adjustments reduce strain now so strength and confidence can return more smoothly later.

Most of these changes don't announce when they're no longer needed. Distances begin to feel shorter. Transitions feel easier. Furniture slowly moves back without a clear turning point. The home returns to its usual rhythm as tolerance improves.

Thinking of preparation this way keeps it from becoming heavy or symbolic. It's not about building a recovery environment. It's about giving your body a quieter, simpler place to move through a demanding phase.

When the space works with you instead of against you, recovery takes up less attention. That leaves more room for rest and patience, and allows progress to unfold without being forced.

A Home That Asks Less of You

When people look back on this phase, they rarely remember specific setups or arrangements. What they remember is whether the days felt manageable.

The homes that work best during early recovery aren't the most prepared. They're the ones that asked the least. Fewer decisions. Fewer adjustments. Less effort spent getting from one moment to the next.

That kind of environment doesn't look special. It feels familiar. It lets you rest without negotiating your surroundings and move without planning every step.

Home preparation doesn't need to be thorough to be effective. It just needs to make daily life a little easier while your energy is low.

When the space supports you quietly, recovery has room to settle. And that's usually enough.

PART TWO

THE FIRST DAYS: WHAT HAPPENS AFTER SURGERY

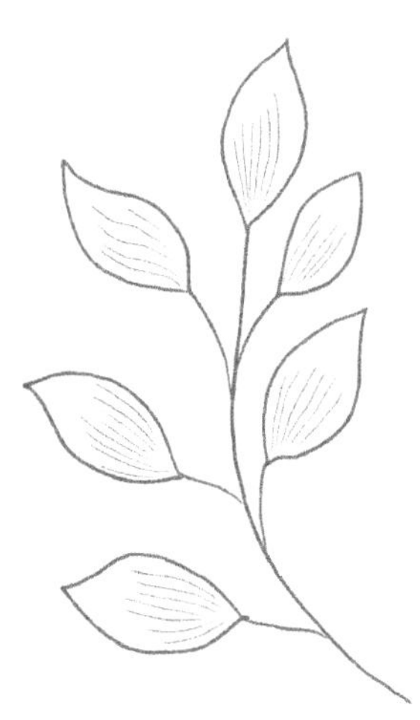

6

The First 72 Hours

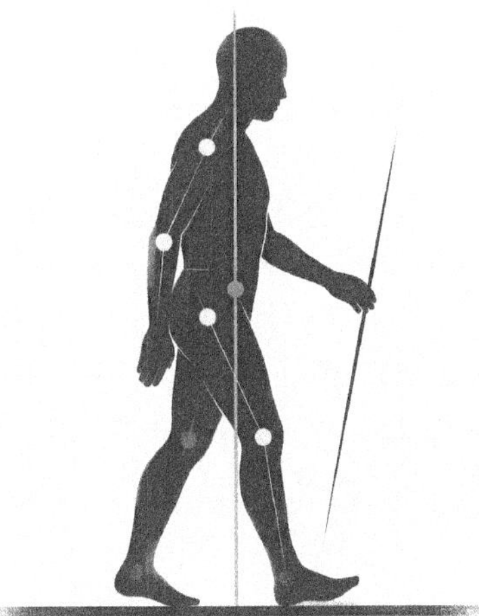

The first hours after surgery rarely match what people imagine. They tend to be quiet, fragmented, and slightly disorienting rather than dramatic. Awareness comes and goes. Time feels uneven. Sensations arrive in pieces instead of forming a clear picture.

This happens because the nervous system is still recalibrating after anesthesia and surgical stress. Signals from the body are dampened, delayed, or partially blocked. What you notice instead is a mix of pressure, warmth, stiffness, or heaviness without a clear center.

Many people expect pain to dominate right away. Often it doesn't. Medications, residual anesthesia, and adrenaline blunt sharp sensations early on. What stands out more is fogginess and a narrowed focus. You're aware of your body, but not in detail. You're present, but not fully oriented.

Clarity returns gradually, not all at once. Awareness comes back in waves, and so does the sense of the joint itself. This early phase is not a signal of how recovery will go. It's a transition period while the body and nervous system reset after a major interruption.

Nothing needs to make sense yet.

Pain That Rises Before It Settles

For many people, pain does not peak immediately after surgery. It builds over time.

In the first hours, medication and leftover anesthesia often keep discomfort muted. As those effects wear off, pain becomes more noticeable. When it rises instead of improving, it can feel alarming, especially if you expected the hardest part to be over.

This pattern is common. Surgical pain behaves differently from the pain you lived with before. It is sharper, more localized, and more reactive to position and movement. It can change quickly, which makes it harder to read.

Swelling is a major driver of this early pain. Fluid accumulates around the joint as part of the inflammatory response. That fluid increases pressure in tissues that were already irritated by surgery. Tightness, throbbing, and a sense of internal pressure often come from this buildup rather than from injury.

Pain also fluctuates because the system is still unstable. Medication timing, rest, small movements, and swelling shifts all interact. One moment may feel manageable. The next may feel intense. That variability does not mean pain control has failed. It reflects a body that has not yet found a steady rhythm.

Expectation plays a role as well. Many people assume pain should steadily improve from the moment surgery ends. When it rises instead, worry can amplify the experience. Early on, the nervous system is especially sensitive to stress.

This phase usually passes as pain becomes more predictable. Peaks soften. Patterns become easier to recognize. That predictability is often the first sign that things are settling, even if pain is still present.

For now, rising pain is not a verdict. It is part of the shift from surgical trauma toward healing.

Fatigue and Mental Fog

Fatigue and Mental Fog

Alongside pain, many people are surprised by how exhausted they feel in the first day or two. This is not ordinary tiredness. It is heavy, sudden, and often out of proportion to how little activity has happened.

Surgery places multiple demands on the body at once. Anesthesia, blood loss, inflammation, and the stress response all draw from the same energy reserves. When those reserves are low, fatigue appears quickly and does not lift with a short rest.

Mental fog often comes with that fatigue. Thinking feels slower. Concentration fades easily. Words may feel just out of reach. This can be unsettling, especially if you are used to being mentally sharp and in control.

These changes reflect how the nervous system prioritizes recovery. Sleep is disrupted. Medications affect attention and memory. The brain narrows its focus to essential tasks and filters out everything else.

That narrowing can feel strange. Your world may shrink to immediate needs—comfort, position, timing, getting from one place to another. Conversations feel shorter. Plans feel distant. This is not withdrawal or disengagement. It is conservation.

Fatigue and fog rarely lift in a straight line. One hour you may feel almost normal. The next, deeply worn out again. That inconsistency is typical early on, not a setback.

As the body stabilizes, energy returns in brief windows. Focus sharpens, then softens again. Over time, those windows widen, and mental clarity becomes more reliable.

Emotional Sensitivity

In the first days after surgery, emotions often feel closer to the surface than expected. Small frustrations can feel larger. Tears or irritability may appear without a clear reason. This can be confusing, especially if you usually handle stress well.

Several things converge at once. Pain medication and anesthesia affect emotional regulation. Sleep is fragmented. Inflammation places the body under sustained stress. At the same time, independence is limited, and reliance on others increases. Together, these factors lower the threshold for emotional reactions.

These responses are not logical or consistent. Relief that surgery is over can exist alongside sudden sadness. Gratitude for help can coexist with irritation. These contrasts do not cancel each other out, and they do not signal regret or weakness.

Another reason emotions surface is the absence of normal distractions. Routines pause. Activity is restricted. Quiet stretches become longer. Feelings that would usually pass unnoticed have more space to appear.

This phase is usually temporary. As pain becomes more predictable, sleep improves, and autonomy increases, emotional intensity tends to soften on its own. It does not require analysis or correction.

Mood shifts during this stage reflect a system under load rather than a problem with recovery itself.

Fluctuating Swelling and Stiffness

Swelling in the first days after surgery rarely stays the same from hour to hour. It increases, settles, then rises again. That movement can make the joint feel unpredictable.

This happens because the inflammatory response is still active. Fluid moves in and out of the tissues based on position, circulation, and recent activity. Even small changes can alter how tight or heavy the joint feels.

Stiffness often follows the same pattern. After resting, the joint may feel rigid or resistant. After gentle movement, it may feel looser for a while, then tighten again as swelling shifts. These changes reflect fluid pressure and tissue sensitivity, not loss of motion.

Swelling can also affect nearby areas. The limb may feel fuller above or below the joint. Skin may feel stretched or warmer than usual. These sensations often change throughout the day, which can be unsettling if you expect steady improvement.

Early swelling tends to feel worse before it improves. As the body regulates fluid more effectively, these swings usually become smaller and less frequent.

For now, variability is part of the process. A joint that feels different from one hour to the next is behaving as expected in the early phase.

Interpreting Early Signals

In the first days after surgery, the body sends a lot of information at once. Sensations feel louder and harder to interpret because nothing feels familiar yet.

What usually matters most is pattern rather than intensity. Sensations that fluctuate—sharp pain with certain movements, sudden stiffness after resting, pressure that comes and goes—are common in early recovery. They reflect swelling shifts and tissue sensitivity more than damage.

What tends to stand out when something needs attention is persistence. A symptom that steadily worsens without easing. Swelling that keeps increasing instead of settling between periods of rest. Discomfort that does not change at all despite shifts in position or time. These experiences feel different because they move in one direction.

Asymmetry is another common source of concern. One side feels heavier. One hour feels better than the next. Early recovery is uneven by nature. Balance and symmetry return gradually, not day by day.

Many people worry about causing harm. A painful step. A movement that feels wrong. Early discomfort usually reflects irritation rather than injury. Sensation often lags behind what tissues can tolerate, especially when swelling is present.

What helps most is watching trends across the day instead of judging single moments. Does pain settle between spikes. Does recovery after effort happen a little faster than it did before. These quiet shifts carry more meaning than any one sensation.

In the first days, much of what you feel is expected noise. Learning to let that noise exist without reacting to every signal reduces mental strain at a time when energy is limited.

7

Pain, Swelling, and Medication

After surgery, many people expect pain to follow a simple arc—strong at first, then steadily easing. When it doesn't behave that way, it can feel unsettling. What's happening is less about something going wrong and more about several systems adjusting at the same time.

Early pain is variable by nature. Swelling shifts through the day. Positioning changes pressure inside the joint. Medication rises and falls in effect. Even time of day matters. As a result, you might feel fairly comfortable one hour and noticeably worse the next, without a clear cause. That swing is common in the early weeks.

Part of the unpredictability comes from the nervous system. After surgery, it stays more alert than usual. Signals that would normally fade into the background are amplified. This doesn't mean damage is increasing. It means the system is still on guard, reacting quickly to changes in load, posture, or fatigue.

Another piece is timing. Pain often lags behind activity. It may rise after rest, then ease with gentle movement, or flare briefly after doing more and settle later. If you judge progress by how you feel in a single moment, that back-and-forth can look like regression even when recovery is moving forward.

Attention plays a role too. When pain doesn't match expectations, focus sharpens. Small changes feel larger. That heightened awareness can make normal fluctuations feel alarming, especially before patterns become familiar.

Consistency usually arrives later, once swelling decreases and daily routines stabilize. Before then, improvement often shows up as pain settling between spikes and feeling more manageable overall—not as a smooth, steady drop.

Early recovery isn't measured hour to hour. It's measured by whether symptoms calm again after they rise and whether the overall load becomes easier to live with across days.

When Pain Rises After Activity — and Why That's Not a Setback

One of the most confusing parts of early recovery is feeling worse after doing something that seemed reasonable. You move more, sit up longer, or have a better day—and later, pain increases. It can feel like proof that you did too much or moved backward.

What's often happening is a delayed response. Healing tissues and a sensitive nervous system don't always react in real time. They register load slowly. The joint may tolerate activity in the moment, then respond hours later with soreness, stiffness, or swelling. That delay can make cause and effect hard to read.

This kind of reactivity is common early on. Tissues are still adjusting to new stresses. Muscles fatigue more quickly. The joint hasn't built consistent tolerance yet. A response later in the day doesn't mean the activity was harmful. It usually means the system noticed the load after the fact.

Pain rising after activity is different from pain that keeps climbing without settling. In early recovery, it often peaks and then eases again with rest. That pattern—react, then calm—is a sign that the system is working through exposure, not failing at it.

Another reason this feels discouraging is timing. Good days often come first in function. You may move more easily or feel steadier before pain becomes predictable. When discomfort follows that improvement, it can feel like progress was imaginary. In reality, function often leads, and symptoms follow more slowly.

It helps to think in terms of recovery windows rather than single events. If pain rises but then settles again, the system is learning. If it returns to baseline by the next day, that's not lost ground. It's information about tolerance.

Setbacks usually announce themselves clearly. They persist. They don't calm with rest. Temporary soreness after activity rarely fits that pattern, even when it's uncomfortable.

Why Function Often Improves Before Pain Settles

Many people expect pain to be the first thing to improve. When it isn't, it can feel discouraging, especially if movement or daily tasks are getting easier at the same time. This mismatch is common in early recovery.

Function and pain are not controlled by the same systems. Strength, coordination, and confidence can return while tissues are still sensitive. You may walk more steadily, stand up more easily, or manage daily tasks with less effort even though discomfort lingers. That doesn't mean the improvement is fragile. It means different parts of recovery move at different speeds.

Early on, the body often prioritizes stability and movement patterns. Muscles relearn how to support the joint. Balance improves. The joint feels more reliable. Pain, on the other hand, is influenced by inflammation, swelling, and nervous system sensitivity, all of which take longer to settle.

This can create a confusing experience. You do more because you can, then pain reminds you that healing isn't finished. It can feel like the body is sending mixed messages. In reality, it's giving layered ones. Capability is increasing. Tolerance is still catching up.

Pain during this phase is often reactive rather than limiting. It shows up after activity instead of stopping you during it. That distinction matters. Pain that allows movement and then eases with rest behaves differently from pain that blocks movement outright.

Progress in this stage often looks like doing more with similar or slightly less discomfort, not doing the same with no pain. Over time, as swelling decreases and sensitivity calms, pain begins to align more closely with function.

Until then, it's common for improvement to feel incomplete. Function leads. Comfort follows later.

Making Sense of "Good Days" and "Bad Days"

Early recovery rarely settles into a steady rhythm right away. Instead, days tend to vary. One day feels easier. The next feels heavier, slower, or more uncomfortable. When that happens, it's easy to assume something has gone wrong.

Day-to-day variability is usually a reflection of load, not damage. Small differences add up. Sleep quality, how long you were upright, how activity was spaced, even stress or concentration demands can change how the system feels the next day. These factors don't announce themselves clearly, but the body responds to them.

The nervous system also plays a role. When it's still vigilant, it reacts strongly to accumulation. A day that goes well may quietly push the system close to its current tolerance. The following day, symptoms rise even if you do less. That lag can make the harder day feel unearned or unfair.

Good days are not a preview of how you should feel from now on. They're snapshots of what's possible when conditions line up. Bad days are not failures. They're feedback about current limits. Neither one defines the direction of recovery on its own.

Progress shows up in patterns across several days. Bad days shorten. Good days become more frequent. The swing between them narrows. Pain settles faster after it rises. These shifts are easy to miss if attention stays fixed on single days.

When recovery is non-linear, trends matter more than moments. Understanding that helps reduce the sense that you're constantly starting over.

When Fluctuations Are Normal — and When They're Not

Most changes in pain and swelling early on are expected. They rise and fall. They respond to rest. They shift with position or time of day. Learning to live with that background noise is part of this phase.

What usually deserves attention is not intensity, but pattern. Normal fluctuations tend to move in both directions. They spike, then settle. They feel reactive. When something isn't right, symptoms often change in one direction only.

Pain that increases day after day without easing. Swelling that builds and doesn't reduce between rests. Warmth or redness that spreads instead of stabilizing. These patterns stand out because they don't behave like the usual ups and downs.

Another difference is responsiveness. Expected symptoms still respond, at least somewhat, to the things that usually help. When pain stops settling at all, or begins interfering more with basic function over time, that's worth noticing.

Brief sharp sensations, soreness after activity, or stiffness that eases with movement are common early on. They can feel alarming, but they usually fit the pattern of a system that's still sensitive rather than injured.

Distinguishing between fluctuation and signal gets easier with time. As routines stabilize, the noise quiets. What remains is clearer, and easier to interpret.

For now, watching trends rather than moments offers the most reliable perspective. When something truly needs attention, it tends to persist and announce itself without constant checking.

Reading Progress Without Using Pain as the Score

Pain is the most obvious signal after surgery, so it's natural to use it as the main measure of how things are going. The problem is that pain is also the most reactive signal. It responds quickly to fatigue, stress, swelling, and timing. That makes it a noisy indicator in the early weeks.

Progress often shows up elsewhere first. The joint settles faster after irritation. Discomfort stays within a narrower range. You spend less time bracing or guarding. Daily tasks require less mental effort. These shifts can happen even while pain still fluctuates.

Another sign of progress is predictability. Early on, pain feels random. Later, patterns begin to form. You start to recognize what leads to a harder evening or a better morning. When symptoms make more sense, they usually feel more manageable, even before they're consistently lower.

It also helps to notice recovery across days rather than within them. A rough afternoon doesn't erase a calmer night. A sore day doesn't cancel a week that was easier overall. When pain is the only score, these gains are easy to miss.

Pain matters, but it isn't the full story. In early recovery, it often lags behind improvement instead of leading it. When you widen the lens, progress becomes easier to see—even when symptoms still rise and fall.

Why "Setbacks" Often Aren't Setbacks

When recovery feels uneven, it's easy to label any harder day as a setback. The word itself suggests lost ground. In early recovery, most of these moments don't fit that meaning.

What's usually happening is exposure followed by response. You do a bit more. The system reacts. Then it settles again. This cycle is how tolerance builds. Without some response, there's no information for the body to adapt to.

True setbacks tend to behave differently. They change the baseline. Pain doesn't return to where it was. Swelling stays elevated. Function drops and doesn't rebound. These shifts are noticeable because they persist, not because they're intense.

Most early "setbacks" are temporary spikes that resolve with time and rest. They can feel discouraging, but they don't erase progress. In fact, they often happen right after a small gain—when function improves before tolerance fully catches up.

Another reason these moments feel heavy is expectation. When you start to feel better, you expect that direction to continue. A reversal, even a brief one, feels more significant than it would earlier on. That emotional weight doesn't reflect actual damage.

Recovery in the early weeks is about calibration. The system tests limits, reacts, and adjusts. That process looks messy from the inside. From the outside, it's typical.

Understanding this doesn't make harder days pleasant. It makes them easier to place. They're part of learning where the edges are, not signs that you've gone backward.

When Things Start to Feel More Stable

Early recovery is defined by change. Sensations shift. Responses feel delayed. Good and bad days trade places without much warning. That phase doesn't last forever, but it also doesn't end suddenly.

Stability usually arrives gradually. Swelling decreases. Daily routines become more predictable. The nervous system stays calmer for longer stretches. Pain still appears, but it behaves more consistently. It settles faster. It surprises you less.

This shift often happens quietly. There isn't a clear moment when recovery feels "normal." Instead, you notice fewer sharp swings. Fewer days that feel like a reset. More stretches where symptoms stay within a familiar range.

Until that point, inconsistency is not a sign of failure. It's a sign that healing systems are still adjusting. Early recovery is a period of sorting and recalibrating, not steady output.

As the body finds its footing, progress becomes easier to recognize. Variability narrows. Confidence grows. Pain begins to follow function instead of interrupting it.

That change is what marks the next phase—not the absence of discomfort, but the return of steadiness.

Holding the Whole Picture Together

In the early weeks, recovery can feel hard to interpret because the signals don't line up neatly. Pain rises and falls. Function improves unevenly. Good days don't always stack, and harder days arrive without warning. None of that means recovery is failing.

What matters most at this stage is direction, not smoothness. Symptoms that react and then settle. Function that gradually expands even when discomfort lingers. Variability that narrows over time. These are the signs the system is adjusting, even when it doesn't feel calm yet.

When you understand that recovery is non-linear, uneven days stop carrying the same weight. They become part of the pattern rather than interruptions to it. Pain becomes one signal among many, not the final verdict on how things are going.

At this point, confusion is common. So is doubt. Neither means you're behind. It means you're still in the phase where the body is learning how to respond again.

Stability comes later. For now, uneven progress is still progress.

8

Moving for the First Time

Early movement after surgery often brings a kind of uncertainty that feels bigger than the motion itself. You can stand. The joint supports you. And yet confidence doesn't arrive at the same time. That gap can feel unsettling, even when nothing is actually wrong.

This reaction is common because standing and walking depend on quick, familiar signals that haven't fully returned yet. Swelling dulls sensation. Muscles may react a little late or a little too strongly. The nervous system stays cautious while it gathers new information. What you're noticing isn't weakness—it's a system that hasn't finished recalibrating its sense of safety.

Because of that, early movement often happens in stages. You prepare. You pause. You move. That deliberate pace can make everything feel fragile, even when the joint itself is stable. The sense of exposure usually comes from uncertainty rather than pain.

What matters here is the pattern, not the moment. If standing and walking are possible with support, and the experience slowly becomes more predictable with repetition, that trend usually reflects normal adjustment. Confidence often trails physical ability, sometimes by days.

It's also typical for steadiness to vary. One attempt may feel easier. The next may feel awkward again. That back-and-forth reflects a nervous system testing limits, not a problem developing.

Unsteady doesn't mean unsafe. It usually means unfamiliar. As repetition continues, signals sharpen, timing improves, and movement begins to feel less demanding—often without a clear turning point.

When Fear Shows Up More Than Pain

In the first days of movement, fear often carries more weight than discomfort. Even when pain is well controlled, hesitation can appear quietly—before a step, during a transfer, or when shifting weight. That reaction can feel confusing, especially if you expected pain to be the main obstacle.

This fear usually grows out of uncertainty rather than damage. For a long time before surgery, pain taught your body to be careful. Certain movements were avoided. Others were guarded. Those protective habits don't disappear just because the joint has been replaced. They tend to linger as caution, even when the structure itself is sound.

Altered feedback plays a role as well. Swelling, healing tissue, and medication change how movement feels. When signals are muted or delayed, the nervous system fills the gap with restraint, slowing things down until it can better predict what will happen next.

Fear often rises and falls. A short walk that goes smoothly may ease it. A sore afternoon can bring it back. That fluctuation is typical early on and doesn't mean progress has reversed. It reflects a system still deciding what it can trust.

What matters more than a single moment of hesitation is the overall direction. When movement keeps happening and nothing harmful follows, fear usually softens on its own. Experience carries more weight than reassurance.

Fear doesn't mean fragility. It means your system is adjusting to a joint that behaves differently than the one it learned to protect. As reactions become more consistent, fear tends to quiet—not because it's forced away, but because it's no longer needed as much.

When Movement Feels Hard Even Though It's Safe

Early on, there's often a disconnect between what you've been told is safe and how movement actually feels. You may know a motion is allowed, even encouraged, and still feel resistance the moment you try it. That mismatch can make people question their judgment.

This happens because the body and instructions operate on different timelines. After surgery, swelling increases pressure in and around the joint. Muscles tighten to protect it. The nervous system stays alert. All of this adds effort to movement, even when nothing is being strained or damaged.

Timing matters too. Muscles don't yet coordinate the way they used to. Some respond slowly. Others jump in too quickly. That uneven timing can make simple actions—standing, stepping, sitting—feel clumsy or tiring, even when basic strength is there.

Because effort feels high, it's easy to assume something is wrong. Most of the time, it's a sign that coordination hasn't settled yet. Early recovery depends less on strength and more on the system relearning how to work together smoothly.

What matters is how this changes with repetition. Movements that feel heavy or awkward at first often begin to require less attention and less effort over time, even if discomfort hasn't fully resolved. That shift usually reflects improving coordination, not increased tolerance for pain.

Hard doesn't mean harmful. Early on, it usually reflects caution, swelling, and unfamiliar timing rather than risk. As those factors ease, movement tends to feel more proportional to the task itself.

When Ordinary Movements Stop Feeling Automatic

After surgery, everyday actions often lose their ease. Sitting down, standing up, turning, or taking a step may suddenly require attention. That change can feel unsettling, especially when you expected recovery to be about returning to normal rather than rethinking each move.

What's happening is adjustment, not loss. The joint moves differently now. Muscles that once worked around pain are changing roles. Sensation is altered by swelling and healing tissue, and the nervous system needs time to update its internal reference points.

Early movement often comes in pieces. You think through steps that used to flow. You move more slowly. You pause and reset. This isn't overthinking—it's integration. Each repetition gives the system clearer information about what's possible and what feels safe.

Variability is part of this phase. A movement may feel easier one day and awkward the next. That swing doesn't mean progress has disappeared. It reflects the system testing and refining new patterns.

What matters is the direction over time. When ordinary movements keep happening, even imperfectly, they tend to require less attention. Actions begin to link together more smoothly, without deliberate planning each step.

Ordinary motion becomes ordinary again through experience, not effort. As the body gathers consistent feedback, it gradually stops asking so many questions, and movement fades back into the background.

When Sensations Change Without Getting Worse

Not all recovery signals announce themselves by getting stronger. Some feel unsettling because they change in quality instead. A new tightness. A different kind of ache. A sense of pressure where there wasn't one before. These shifts can feel more concerning than steady discomfort.

This happens because healing doesn't move in a straight line. Swelling redistributes. Tissues stiffen and soften at different rates. As activity changes, the joint and surrounding muscles respond in new ways. For a time, the nervous system can also become more sensitive before it settles, making sensations feel sharper or more noticeable.

What often causes worry is the surprise. A sensation that wasn't there yesterday appears today, even though nothing obvious has changed. In early recovery, change by itself doesn't always signal a problem. It often reflects a system adapting to new demands.

The pattern matters more than the moment. Sensations that shift but stay linked to activity, time of day, or fatigue usually fit within normal adjustment. Those that ease, even gradually, with rest or repetition tend to follow that pattern as well.

What deserves closer attention is a change that steadily narrows what you can do over several days, rather than one that fluctuates. Recovery signals often move around before they settle. Problems tend to press in one direction.

Changing sensations can feel unsettling because they're unfamiliar, not because they're dangerous. As healing continues and responses become more predictable, those shifts usually lose their edge, and their meaning becomes clearer with time.

When Progress Feels Inconsistent

Many people expect improvement to feel steady. When it doesn't, the inconsistency itself can raise concern. One day movement feels easier. The next day stiffness, soreness, or hesitation returns. That swing can make it hard to tell whether recovery is actually moving forward.

This pattern is common because several systems are adjusting at the same time. Inflammation rises and falls through the day. Muscles fatigue before they regain endurance. The nervous system reacts to new demands, settles, then reacts again. None of that follows a straight line.

What often creates worry is focusing on a single point in time. How you feel in the afternoon may look very different from how you felt in the morning. A walk that felt manageable yesterday may feel heavier today without a clear reason. Taken alone, those moments can look like setbacks.

Trends tell a clearer story. When harder days are followed by days that feel similar or slightly easier, that usually reflects adaptation rather than decline. When the range of what you can do slowly expands—even if comfort lags behind—that pattern often matters more than daily variability.

In early recovery, inconsistency is often a sign that the system is being challenged and learning, not that it's failing. True problems tend to reduce capacity steadily. Normal recovery tends to wobble as it moves forward.

Progress doesn't always announce itself clearly. Sometimes it shows up as a difficult day that isn't quite as limiting as the last one, or as recovery that comes a little faster after rest. Those quieter shifts usually carry more meaning than any single uncomfortable moment.

When Patterns Matter More Than Sensations

As recovery continues, it's easy to start paying close attention to every signal. A twinge. A pause. A new feeling. That focus often comes from wanting to protect the joint, but it can make normal fluctuations feel more significant than they are.

The body doesn't heal in isolated moments. It responds over hours and days. Swelling shifts. Sensitivity rises and falls. Energy changes with sleep, activity, and stress. When you look too closely at any single sensation, you lose the context that gives it meaning.

Patterns restore that context. Noticing how something behaves over time—rather than how it feels right now—usually offers clearer information. Does a sensation ease after rest? Does movement become more predictable across the day? Does recovery after activity gradually improve? Those trends tend to matter more than brief discomfort or hesitation.

This doesn't mean ignoring concerns. It means letting them settle into perspective. Most normal recovery signals soften, move, or repeat without tightening their grip. Signals that deserve attention tend to narrow options rather than fluctuate.

Many people find that once they stop checking constantly, their sense of how things are going actually improves. Not because sensations disappear, but because the background noise quiets enough for real change to stand out.

Learning to watch the pattern is part of recovery itself. It allows you to rest mentally while the body does its work, and over time, that wider view often replaces the urge to analyze every feeling.

When Trust Starts Replacing Constant Checking

As this phase continues, something subtle often shifts. You still notice sensations, but they no longer demand immediate interpretation. The joint feels present without feeling threatening, and movement happens with less commentary in your head.

This doesn't mean everything feels good. It means your system has gathered enough experience to place sensations in context. Swelling, stiffness, or effort may still appear, but they fit into patterns you recognize. Familiar signals lose their urgency.

Trust builds quietly this way. Not through a single reassuring moment, but through many ordinary ones where nothing needs fixing. You move. You rest. You recover. And the outcome becomes predictable enough to reduce constant evaluation.

At this point, concern grows more selective. You notice when something truly changes direction, rather than reacting to every fluctuation. That selectivity isn't complacency—it's discernment shaped by experience.

Recovery doesn't settle when sensations disappear. It settles when they stop running the process, and you no longer have to ask each time whether what you're feeling means something is wrong.

◆○◆

By this point, you don't need to interpret every sensation to know how things are going. You've begun to see which signals tend to settle, which ones fluctuate, and which patterns actually deserve attention. That understanding doesn't remove uncertainty, but it changes how much space it takes up. As recovery moves forward, this quieter way of noticing becomes part of daily life—often without you realizing it.

PART THREE

RECOVERY, PHASE BY PHASE

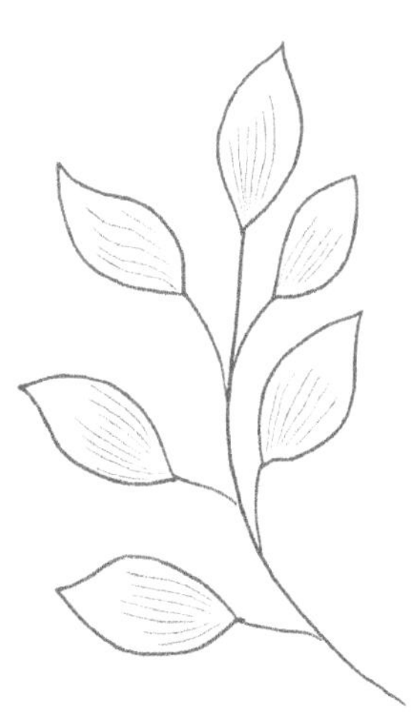

9

Weeks 1–2: Just Getting Through the Day

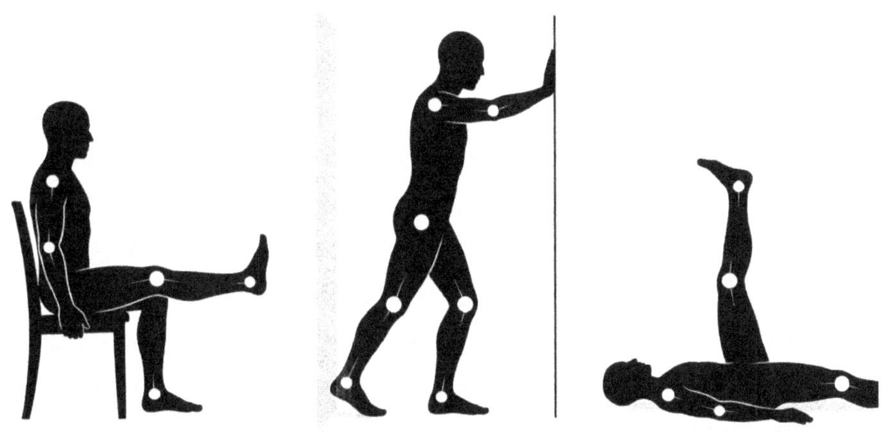

In the first couple of weeks after surgery, many people are caught off guard by how much effort an ordinary day requires. Not a full schedule. Not a demanding set of tasks. Just getting up, washing, eating, and moving between rooms can feel like it uses everything you have.

This creates a particular kind of fatigue. It is deeper than sleepiness and heavier than muscle tiredness. By afternoon, you may feel as if your system has already spent its reserve, even though the day has been quiet on the surface.

Part of this comes from healing itself. Your body is running a constant repair process, managing inflammation and reorganizing tissue. That work draws energy all day long, whether you feel it happening or not. Less energy is left over for movement, thinking, or decision-making.

Another part is attention. In this phase, very little is automatic. Each movement takes focus. Each transition requires planning. Even simple choices carry more weight. That steady mental effort adds to physical fatigue, even when you have not done much.

As a result, the day often breaks into fragments. You do something small, then need to pause. You begin an activity, then stop sooner than expected. This can feel unsettling if you are used to pushing through tiredness. Early recovery does not respond well to that approach.

Needing frequent rest at this stage does not mean you are weak or unprepared. It reflects a system operating at survival level, directing most of its resources toward healing and stability rather than ease or efficiency.

Why the Fatigue Feels Out of Proportion

By this point, many people stop asking why things hurt and start asking why they feel so wiped out. Pain may be more predictable than it was in the first days, yet energy feels unreliable and limited.

This kind of fatigue is not a sign that recovery is going poorly. Surgery places demand on the whole system, not just the joint. Sleep is disrupted. Appetite shifts. The nervous system stays more alert than usual. Even when the incision looks calm, internal work is still ongoing.

Rest does not always feel restorative yet. You may spend plenty of time lying down and still wake up feeling flat. Early on, the body has not returned to its usual rhythm, so rest helps slowly and unevenly rather than all at once.

There is also the cost of constant adjustment. Your brain is working harder to monitor balance, timing, and confidence with movement. Much of that effort runs in the background, unnoticed until the day catches up with you.

Fatigue in this phase tends to arrive in waves. You might feel reasonably steady in the morning, then hit a wall without much warning. Or you may have one day that feels better, followed by two that feel heavier. That uneven pattern is common, even though it often triggers doubt.

When energy feels scarce, it is easy to interpret exhaustion as failure or lack of progress. In reality, it reflects a system still under load, allocating most of its resources to healing and regulation rather than stamina.

Pain That No Longer Follows the Old Rules

Around this stage, many people notice that pain feels different than it did before surgery. That change can be confusing. You may have expected pain to simply fade, not shift in character.

Before surgery, pain often followed a familiar pattern. It showed up with certain movements and eased with rest. Now it may feel sharper at times, dull or tight at others, or more spread out than you expect. It can appear without a clear trigger and linger longer than seems reasonable.

This does not mean something is wrong. After surgery, pain comes from several sources at once. Healing tissue, lingering swelling, sensitive nerves, and altered movement all send signals. Because these systems are still settling, the messages can feel unfamiliar and inconsistent.

One common concern is pain that shows up later rather than during activity. You may move through something without much trouble, then feel the effects hours later or that night. This often reflects a system that managed the effort in the moment but needed more recovery time afterward.

What unsettles many people is the loss of reference points. The old pain is gone, but the new sensations do not yet make sense. Without a clear pattern, every signal can feel suspicious. Over time, those patterns usually become clearer, even before pain fully eases.

At this point, pain is not a measure of damage or success. It is part of a system recalibrating. Understanding how it behaves tends to develop gradually, alongside steadier energy and more predictable days.

A Full Day That Quietly Drains You

During these weeks, effort is often tied less to what you do and more to how long the day lasts. The morning may begin with some clarity. By midday, everything feels heavier. By evening, even small tasks can feel out of proportion to their size.

This is not just physical tiredness. It is cumulative load. Each transition, each adjustment, each moment of attention adds a small demand. None of them stands out on its own. Together, they steadily drain the system.

What makes this phase hard is that energy rarely disappears all at once. It leaks. You may feel mostly fine, then notice your patience thinning, your movements becoming less precise, or pain feeling louder. That shift often arrives without warning.

Mental fatigue often shows up before physical fatigue. Focus slips. Decisions feel harder. Emotional tolerance narrows. By the end of the day, discomfort may feel more widespread, even if the joint itself is not dramatically worse.

Rest still helps, but not immediately. Once the system is overloaded, it takes time to settle. That delay can make it difficult to connect what you did earlier with how you feel later, adding to the sense that the day is unpredictable.

A day that takes all your energy is not a failed day. At this stage, it reflects a body prioritizing healing and stability over endurance. Over time, the same day will demand less, but that change usually comes quietly, after many days like this.

Where You Are in This Phase

This part of recovery often feels like a holding pattern. The initial shock of surgery has passed, but forward motion is still hard to sense. You are no longer counting hours since the operation, yet the weeks ahead feel distant and abstract.

It helps to understand what this stage is doing. Your system is settling. Pain may still be present, but it is becoming more consistent. Swelling may fluctuate, but it no longer feels chaotic. Fatigue remains central, yet it begins to follow rhythms you can start to recognize.

A lot is happening quietly. The nervous system is easing out of constant alert. The body is testing what it can tolerate without setting off a bigger reaction. Small internal adjustments are taking place without your awareness. None of this feels like progress, but it creates the conditions for it.

This is also when comparison tends to creep in. You may look outward for reassurance because your own signals are still mixed. That urge is understandable. At the same time, this window varies widely from person to person, even among those who had similar procedures.

If you are trying to locate yourself in the process, this is a fair description: you are no longer in crisis, but not yet rebuilding. You are in between. That in-between phase is necessary, even if it feels unproductive.

Getting through the day, even when it takes all your energy, is the work of this stage. The shift toward more stability usually begins before comfort or confidence return. When it does, it tends to arrive quietly, noticed only after it has already started.

The Quiet Shift Beneath the Surface

Toward the end of this early window, something often begins to change, even if you would not describe it as improvement. The days are still demanding, but they feel demanding in a more predictable way. The system reacts less dramatically to small variations.

Pain may still be present. Fatigue is often still the dominant feature. What shifts first is not comfort, but steadiness. A slightly busier morning does not automatically unravel the entire day. Recovery from effort, while still slow, becomes more reliable.

This change is easy to miss because it does not feel like relief. Many people expect the next phase to begin when energy returns or pain drops. More often, it begins when swings become less extreme and the body holds its ground more consistently.

This can create a subtle restlessness. You may sense that something is changing, without being able to point to what it is. That feeling often comes before visible gains, not after them.

The work of these weeks has largely been about settling. As that settling takes hold, the next stage becomes possible. Not suddenly. Not cleanly. But gradually, in ways that tend to make more sense once you are a little further along.

10

Weeks 3–4: The Confusing Stage

Recovery often becomes harder to interpret around this point. Not because nothing is happening, but because change no longer moves in a straight line. You may wake up feeling lighter and more capable, then find that the same joint feels heavier or less cooperative a day or two later.

Earlier on, discomfort had a clear explanation. Everything was new, swollen, and obviously healing. Now that some things have improved, inconsistency feels more unsettling. A harder day raises questions that did not come up before, about whether you misjudged something, did too much, or missed a signal.

What is happening is variability, not reversal. As healing progresses, the body tests slightly wider limits. It tolerates more, then reacts. It adapts, then asks for recovery time. These swings reflect adjustment, not loss of progress.

Improvement at this stage shows up as capacity before it shows up as reliability. You can do more on a good day than you could earlier, even if you cannot do it every day yet. That gap between what is possible and what is consistent is what makes this phase feel confusing.

When Patterns Become Harder to Read

As recovery continues, cause and effect become less obvious. A day that feels manageable in the moment may lead to discomfort later. Another day that starts stiff may loosen as it goes on. Because responses are delayed, it becomes harder to link what you did with how you feel afterward.

Earlier, signals were more immediate. Pain rose with movement and settled with rest. Now the timing is less tidy. Symptoms may appear hours later, or even the next day, which makes interpretation unreliable. You may replay the day, trying to identify a single reason, and come up empty.

There is a simple reason for this shift. Inflammation no longer peaks right away, and the nervous system is still adjusting how quickly it reacts. Load is tolerated differently than before, and feedback arrives out of order. That mismatch creates doubt, even when overall healing is moving forward.

When signals are harder to read, individual days lose their value as indicators. A better day does not confirm that things have turned a corner, and a harder one does not explain what went wrong. The information is there, but it takes longer to organize into a clear picture.

Why Pain Feels Different Now

Pain often becomes harder to interpret once the most obvious signs of surgery begin to fade. It may not be stronger than before, but it behaves differently. Sensations shift, move, or appear at times that feel disconnected from what you just did.

Earlier on, pain followed a clearer logic. Incisions were fresh. Swelling was visible. Discomfort matched what you could see and feel on the surface. As the outside settles, pain that lingers or changes form can feel more concerning, even when healing is still progressing as expected.

One of the biggest changes is timing. Discomfort may show up later rather than right away. Another is variability. A movement that felt fine one day may feel irritating the next. This usually reflects tissues and nerves adjusting their thresholds, not new injury.

Pain at this stage also blends more with fatigue and attention. When sleep is lighter or energy dips, tolerance drops and sensations stand out more. Many people respond by tracking every signal closely, which can make patterns feel even less clear.

Here, pain carries less direct meaning than it did earlier. It is often incomplete feedback from systems that are still settling, rather than a clear message that something is wrong.

When Energy Returns Without Stability

Energy often starts to reappear before it becomes dependable. You may notice a few better hours, a morning that feels more workable, or a stretch of the day that feels closer to normal. These moments stand out because they were largely absent earlier.

What makes this phase tricky is that energy does not stay. It shows up in pieces, then drops off again. When that happens, the contrast feels sharp. Having energy and then losing it is more noticeable than not having it at all.

This happens because recovery restores capacity faster than endurance. Your system can generate more energy than before, but it cannot sustain it yet. Small demands add up quickly, and fatigue arrives sooner than expected.

Energy is also more sensitive now. Sleep quality, stimulation, conversation, or a slightly longer day can drain reserves without much warning. When that drop comes, it can feel like a setback, even though it reflects limits that are still being mapped.

Because energy is unreliable, confidence often dips with it. Feeling capable for part of the day and depleted later makes it harder to trust your own signals. That uncertainty is a defining feature of this stage, not a sign that progress has stalled.

The Mental Load of Self-Monitoring

As recovery becomes less externally structured, more decisions shift onto you. Early on, the day was shaped by clear limits. Rest, medication, and short bouts of activity created a simple framework. Now that some of those boundaries loosen, interpretation takes their place.

You may find yourself checking in constantly. How does this feel? Is that sensation expected? Did I do too much, or not enough? None of these questions is new, but they come up more often because the answers are less clear.

This ongoing self-monitoring carries its own fatigue. It asks for attention at the same time that physical energy is still uneven. When signals are inconsistent and feedback is delayed, even small choices start to feel loaded with consequence.

Overdoing and underdoing can also feel similar here. Both may lead to stiffness, soreness, or tiredness later on. Without immediate feedback, it becomes hard to tell which direction you missed, which feeds doubt rather than clarity.

The mental effort of trying to get it right is part of why this phase often feels harder than earlier weeks. The body may be healing, but the work of interpretation has increased.

Why Confidence Often Drops Despite Progress

By this point, many signs of recovery are present. Daily tasks take less effort. Movement feels less fragile. Pain may be lower overall. Yet confidence often slips rather than grows.

That drop makes sense. Early confidence came from clear rules and visible change. Each small improvement stood out against a backdrop of limitation. Now progress is quieter, while variability is more noticeable.

Confidence also depends on predictability. When good days and harder days alternate without warning, trust erodes. You may hesitate more, even while doing more, because outcomes feel uncertain.

There is often a growing gap between what you can do and how it feels afterward. Activity may be possible, but delayed responses make it harder to judge its cost. Without reliable feedback, confidence has little to anchor to.

This phase can feel mentally heavier than the first weeks for that reason. Progress is real, but it has not yet settled into patterns that feel dependable.

A Phase Defined by Adjustment, Not Clarity

By the end of this stage, many people feel less certain than they did earlier. That can be unsettling, especially if you expected understanding to increase as time passed. Instead, more variables are active at once, and they do not line up cleanly.

You are no longer responding only to surgery. Healing tissue, shifting pain, uneven energy, delayed responses, and rising expectations all interact. When those elements fall out of sync, the overall picture can feel wrong even when progress is present.

This period is less about forward momentum and more about adjustment. The body is testing wider limits and reporting back with mixed signals. That back-and-forth is how tolerance builds, even though it feels inefficient from the inside.

Looking back, there is usually more change than it seems day to day. Pain behaves differently. Fatigue has a different shape. Daily life is still restricted, but less fragile. These shifts are subtle and easy to miss when focus stays on what has not settled yet.

Confusion at this point is not a detour from recovery. It reflects a system in transition, still organizing its responses. As those responses stabilize, clarity usually follows.

11

Weeks 5–8: Slow Progress and New Frustrations

There comes a point in recovery when change no longer feels obvious. Things are not falling apart, but they are not clearly getting better either. Days run more smoothly than before, yet nothing stands out as a win you can point to in the moment.

What often changes first is not comfort, but how smoothly things run. Movements require less planning. Transitions take fewer adjustments. You recover a bit faster after doing something demanding. Because these shifts happen quietly, they are easy to overlook or discount.

Another reason progress feels muted is that it becomes easier to recognize only in hindsight. From one day to the next, everything can feel much the same. Looking back a couple of weeks, there is a difference. That delay between change and awareness makes improvement feel slower than it actually is.

At the same time, different systems improve at different speeds. Movement may be smoother while stiffness lingers. Endurance may increase while soreness still shows up in the morning. This unevenness can create the sense that progress is partial or unstable, even when the overall direction is forward.

Frustration often starts here not because recovery has stalled, but because expectations have shifted. Early on, simply getting through the day felt like enough. Now that daily life is more manageable, the mind looks for clearer reward. When improvement arrives quietly instead, it can feel disappointing.

Progress that no longer calls attention to itself is still progress. Subtle change at this point usually reflects recovery settling, not slipping away.

Aches That Appear Without a Clear Pattern

New or shifting aches often show up in this part of recovery, even when earlier pain has eased. They are not always sharp, and they do not always stay in one place. One day stiffness stands out. Another day it fades, only to return later without an obvious trigger.

That unpredictability can feel discouraging. When something new appears after you thought pain was settling, it is easy to assume something has gone wrong. More often, these sensations reflect a system that is being asked to do more, not one that is being harmed.

The quality of stiffness also tends to change. It may show up more after rest than during movement. It may ease once you get going, then return later in the day. If you expect stiffness to steadily decline as recovery continues, this pattern can be confusing.

Variability is a common feature here. A day that feels workable may be followed by one that feels tight and resistant. That swing does not mean progress is reversing. It usually means load tolerance is still adjusting and has not settled into a reliable rhythm yet.

Fatigue plays a role as well. When energy dips, tolerance drops, and sensations feel louder. The joint itself may not be doing worse, but the system has less buffer to manage demand, so discomfort stands out more.

Aches that come and go in this phase are often part of adjustment rather than injury. The body is relearning how to share load across tissues. That process is uneven, and it rarely feels smooth while it is happening.

Why Gains Are Real but Hard to Feel

Doing more does not always come with the feeling of improvement. By this point, many people have clearly increased their activity compared to earlier weeks, yet feel unsure that much has changed.

One reason is that progress no longer announces itself as relief. Tasks take less mental effort. Recovery after activity is quicker. These shifts reduce strain, but they do not necessarily create comfort, so they are easy to miss.

Another reason is that the internal measuring stick has moved. Early in recovery, small changes felt significant. As daily life becomes more manageable, the bar rises. Improvement that once would have felt meaningful can now seem underwhelming.

There is also a delay in awareness. You often realize something has improved only when it no longer demands attention. That recognition comes after the change has already settled in, which makes progress feel slow even when it is steady.

From a healing standpoint, this phase involves quieter work. Tissues are reorganizing and adapting to repeated use, which happens gradually. The nervous system is also settling, allowing more activity while still keeping signals present. These processes favor stability over dramatic change.

Feeling unimpressed by progress does not mean it is not happening. It means recovery has shifted from survival toward rebuilding, where gains are real but less satisfying to notice.

More Capacity Without Matching Comfort

The day may look fuller now. You spend more time on your feet, move through routines with less hesitation, and engage with normal life more often. What makes this phase difficult is that comfort does not always rise alongside that increase.

There is an understandable expectation that if you can do more, you should feel better doing it. Recovery rarely works that way. Capacity often improves first. Comfort tends to follow later, and at a slower pace.

Part of this lag comes from tissue adaptation. Healing structures are still remodeling and responding to repeated load, which takes time even when basic healing is complete. At the same time, the nervous system remains watchful. It allows more activity but continues to flag it as something to monitor, keeping sensations present.

Symptoms may also shift rather than disappear. Discomfort can feel milder but more frequent, or show up later in the day instead of during activity. Those changes can obscure improvement, even when overall tolerance is higher.

This gap between what you can handle and how it feels to handle it is a common transition. It is uncomfortable, but it is not a dead end. For many people, comfort eventually catches up to capacity without a clear turning point.

If things feel slow but steadier now, that is not a stall. It is consolidation. Recovery is becoming more predictable, even before it becomes easier to live with.

From Swings to Something Steadier

Without a clear moment of change, many people begin to notice that the extremes soften. Harder days still happen, but they do not feel as destabilizing. Better days no longer feel fragile or rare.

This shift is less about improvement speeding up and more about patterns repeating. The body starts responding in familiar ways. You learn what a manageable day feels like and how it differs from one that needs more recovery time.

Consistency arrives as predictability before it arrives as comfort. Stiffness, fatigue, or lingering pain may still be present, but they behave more reliably. That reliability reduces mental load, even when symptoms themselves have not eased much.

From a physiological standpoint, this reflects systems settling. Load tolerance becomes steadier, and the nervous system becomes less reactive. Signals are still there, but they are less surprising.

This steadier ground is the bridge into the next phase of recovery. Progress becomes easier to interpret, not because recovery is finished, but because it no longer feels fragile.

If things feel slow yet more stable now, that is not a plateau. It is the work of these weeks taking hold quietly, setting the stage for greater consistency ahead.

12

Physical Therapy: What Helps and What Doesn't

It's tempting to assume that physical therapy should keep driving visible progress the same way it did at the start. When that momentum fades, doubt often fills the gap. If sessions no longer feel dramatic, it's easy to wonder whether something has gone off track.

What usually changes here is not the usefulness of therapy, but its function. Instead of jump-starting movement, it begins to organize what your body can already handle. The aim is less about adding challenge and more about reducing mixed signals, so effort stops competing with itself.

This phase tends to reward work that leaves you more stable afterward, even if it causes short-lived discomfort. The difference shows up later in the day: easier transitions, less guarding, a calmer sense of movement. Effort that feels productive in the moment but disrupts sleep or drains energy often leads in the opposite direction.

When therapy feels quieter now, that is often a sign of fit rather than failure. Its value shifts toward helping your system settle into patterns that hold up outside the clinic, without needing to announce themselves during the session.

Why "More" Doesn't Automatically Lead Forward

What helps one week can irritate the next, and that contradiction catches many people off guard. There is a strong pull to believe that recovery keeps responding to added effort in a straight line. More intensity, more time, more challenge. It sounds logical, even responsible.

At this stage, the body responds more to tolerance than to determination. It can accept more overall, but only when that load matches how sensitive the system is right now. When demand rises faster than integration, progress often becomes noisier rather than clearer.

This is why effort and benefit stop lining up cleanly. A session that feels demanding can leave you unsettled later, while another that feels almost uneventful may support a steadier day. Without obvious feedback, it's easy to assume the harder option must be the more effective one.

What's happening beneath the surface is adaptation competing with irritation. Helpful work allows the system to adjust without needing to defend itself afterward. Less helpful work borrows from future energy, leaving fatigue, irritability, or lingering soreness that feels out of proportion.

Understanding this usually eases pressure. Progress does not slow because effort becomes more measured. It often becomes more consistent because the body finally has room to absorb what it's being asked to do.

Reading Discomfort Without Overreacting

By now, some level of discomfort is expected, which makes interpretation harder. The question shifts from whether something feels uncomfortable to what that discomfort represents, if anything at all.

Discomfort that supports recovery usually has a clear arc. It appears during or shortly after movement, stays local, and then fades. It doesn't change how you feel overall. You may notice soreness or stiffness, but your mood, energy, and sense of control remain largely intact.

Signals that ask for pause behave differently. They linger, spread, or show up later. Sleep becomes lighter. The next day feels heavier than expected, not just in the joint but across the system. Instead of settling, the reaction accumulates.

This difference is rarely obvious at first. Most people recognize it only after seeing the same pattern repeat. That isn't a missed cue. It's how the system clarifies which inputs it can use and which ones overload it.

In this phase, discomfort alone isn't a reliable scorecard. What matters more is what follows. Over time, those after-effects become a clearer guide than how things felt in the moment.

When Therapy Simplifies Recovery — or Complicates It

Some sessions leave things feeling more organized, even if nothing dramatic happened. Movement later in the day feels steadier. Spikes are fewer. Discomfort may still be present, but it doesn't dominate attention or alter how you move.

Other times, everything feels harder to read afterward. Fatigue lingers. Sleep is disrupted. Symptoms blur together instead of separating into clearer signals. Instead of feeling more confident, you become more cautious.

This difference isn't about doing therapy "right" or wrong. It's about match. When the work fits where your system is that day, therapy reduces uncertainty. When it doesn't, it adds confusion.

The reason is straightforward. A system that is still sensitive reacts strongly to how load is introduced. Even well-intended input can overwhelm if timing or tolerance is off. When the fit is right, similar work can help the body settle rather than stir.

Recognizing this pattern shifts attention away from individual sensations and toward overall response, which is often the clearest signal available at this stage.

Why Progress Often Shows Up Away From the Clinic

It can be surprising when some of your better days don't follow therapy sessions at all. You may feel steadier on days without appointments, or notice improvements during ordinary activities rather than after focused work.

This doesn't mean therapy has stopped helping. It usually means your body integrates change on its own timeline. Sessions introduce exposure and direction. Daily life is where those inputs are tested without pressure or close observation.

Outside the clinic, movement is often less deliberate. You're not monitoring every sensation or bracing for response. When attention softens, the nervous system often follows, and movement becomes easier and more natural.

There's also the role of recovery time. Therapy adds demand, even when it's appropriate. The benefit may not show up until the system has space to absorb that input. When that space is present, improvement can feel quiet but durable.

At this stage, progress doesn't need to announce where it came from to count. If days feel more manageable and movement feels less effortful, therapy is often doing its work in the background, even when the clinic isn't where change is most obvious.

When Trust Becomes Part of the Process

Here, how therapy feels often matters as much as what happens during a session. Trust starts to play a larger role, not as an abstract idea, but as a practical part of recovery. You're no longer just doing the work. You're sensing whether the process fits you.

Many people carry quiet tension into this phase. They want guidance, but they also worry about being pushed into something that will cost them days afterward. That hesitation is understandable. Your body is more capable now, yet setbacks feel more expensive.

Trust grows when your responses are taken seriously. When a harder day leads to adjustment rather than dismissal. When discomfort is explored, not brushed aside or framed as something you simply need to tolerate. Over time, that responsiveness reduces the mental load around sessions.

When trust is missing, therapy can feel heavier than it needs to be. You may brace during work, second-guess afterward, or hold back information to avoid being seen as difficult. None of that helps recovery settle.

When trust is present, therapy tends to simplify rather than complicate this stage. It becomes a shared process of noticing patterns and adjusting together, with the focus staying on helping your body function more reliably, not on proving effort or endurance.

13

Setbacks, Bad Days, and Fear of Going Backward

A bad day carries more weight once progress has begun. Earlier on, discomfort was expected and constant. Now that you have seen improvement, a sudden harder day feels loaded with meaning. It can seem as if something fragile has been lost.

These days often start without a clear trigger. You wake up stiffer. Movement feels less smooth. Pain takes up more attention. Nothing dramatic has happened, yet the tone of the day feels wrong. That contrast alone can create unease before you have done very much.

Memory plays a role here. You can clearly recall better days now, and that comparison sharpens disappointment. When everything was difficult, variation mattered less. Once things improve, variation starts to feel personal, as if the body is sending mixed messages.

What changes on a bad day is not what you have gained, but how much of it is accessible. The capacity you have built is still there. It is simply less available when the system is tired, irritated, or running low on reserve.

Many of these days reflect accumulated load rather than a single misstep. Several decent days in a row, lighter sleep, or background stress can quietly narrow tolerance. When the buffer runs thin, the body signals it.

This is often the first point where fear of going backward appears. That fear does not mean you are regressing. It means recovery has reached a stage where fluctuation feels threatening. Learning to read that signal without assigning it too much meaning is part of what comes next.

Why Setbacks Often Follow Better Days

Progress often triggers the very thing that feels most discouraging. A stretch of smoother days can lead to a setback that seems to arrive out of nowhere. The timing feels wrong, as if improvement should protect you from feeling worse.

What usually changes on better days is not just comfort, but demand. You move more freely. You stay upright longer. You engage more with daily life. None of this feels excessive in the moment, because it fits within what you can do.

The body often allows that increase before it fully registers the cost. Tissues respond to load with a delay. Inflammation can rise hours or even a day later, once the system starts to process what it handled. When recovery time does not quite match the increase in demand, symptoms show up after the fact.

That delayed response is why setbacks rarely feel dramatic. They appear as stiffness that lingers, pain that feels louder, or fatigue that arrives sooner than expected. These changes are signals of reactivity, not signs that healing has reversed.

Seen in this light, a setback after better days is not a contradiction. It is feedback that the system used the capacity it has been building. The capacity itself does not disappear because the response arrived late.

Fear That Progress Is Slipping Away

Fear tends to rise faster than symptoms. When a harder day appears, the first worry is often not about pain itself, but about what it might mean. The thought is immediate: maybe this is the start of going backward.

That fear usually shows up only after progress has become real. Earlier on, everything was uncertain, so there was little to lose. Once improvement exists, it can feel fragile. A bad day then reads like proof that the gains were temporary.

What gets missed in that moment is where progress actually lives. It is not stored in how you feel today. It is stored in capacity built over time. A flare limits access to that capacity for a while, but it does not erase it.

The nervous system adds another layer. When threat detection is high, sensations are amplified. Stiffness feels sharper. Fatigue feels heavier. The body becomes harder to interpret when fear is layered on top of normal signals.

This is why people often react in opposite ways on bad days. Some test limits to check if they are still capable. Others pull back completely, worried that any movement will make things worse. Both reactions come from uncertainty, not from what the body is actually doing.

Fear of slipping backward does not mean you are. It means recovery matters now. As the same pattern repeats—better days, harder days, then steadier ground—that fear usually loses its grip before the symptoms do.

How the Body Signals Overload

Overload rarely announces itself while you are doing more. It shows up later, once the system has time to react. Pain lingers longer than usual. Sleep feels lighter or more broken. Fatigue arrives earlier and feels heavier than it should.

These signals are often subtle. They do not feel like warnings, which is why they are easy to dismiss or misread. When attention is focused on holding progress, early signs of strain can slip by unnoticed.

Mental changes are common as well. Irritability increases. Focus drops. Small frustrations feel outsized. These shifts are easy to blame on mood, but they often track closely with physical strain.

Timing adds to the confusion. Because the response is delayed, the cause is no longer obvious. That makes overload feel random. Often, the pattern only becomes clear in hindsight.

As this pattern becomes familiar, setbacks lose some of their shock. Overload starts to read less like a problem and more like information. That shift alone reduces fear, even when symptoms flare.

What a Setback Actually Means

By the time setbacks start to worry you, recovery has already moved past its most fragile phase. That changes what a setback represents. Earlier on, a bad turn could feel alarming because everything was still new and unstable. Now, a setback usually means something else.

Most setbacks reflect a short-term mismatch between demand and re-covery, not a loss of healing. The system took on more than it could comfortably absorb and responded by narrowing tolerance for a while. That response can feel intense, but it is protective rather than harmful.

The time scale is easy to misread. Capacity builds over weeks. A flare plays out over days. When discomfort spikes, it can feel as if weeks of progress disappeared overnight. In reality, access to that capacity changed, not the capacity itself.

Setbacks at this stage are often partial. One area flares while others remain steady. Pain may increase while movement stays similar, or fatigue rises without a loss of confidence. These mixed signals are signs that recovery is layered, not all-or-nothing.

Over time, setbacks also tend to shorten. Even when they feel sharp at first, the system usually settles more quickly than it did earlier. That shortening can be easy to miss if attention stays fixed on discomfort alone.

Seen this way, a setback is not a verdict. It is feedback. Something to notice, not something to fear, as the body continues adjusting and recalibrating.

What's Normal — and What's Not

As recovery settles into a steadier rhythm, attention often shifts from how much something hurts to what each sensation seems to mean. Familiar discomfort is easier to place. New or changing signals stand out more sharply, not because they are severe, but because they interrupt a sense of predictability that is just beginning to form.

Many experiences at this stage still fall within a wide, expected range. Ongoing soreness, stiffness after rest, swelling that comes and goes, or aching later in the day usually reflect continued adaptation rather than a problem with healing. What makes them hard to live with is less their presence and more their timing and inconsistency.

Unpredictability often carries more weight than intensity. A sensation that appears without an obvious cause, lingers longer than expected, and then fades can feel more unsettling than steady discomfort. The mind looks for rules, and recovery rarely offers simple ones.

It is also common for symptoms to change their character over time. Sharp pain may soften but become more constant. Soreness may give way to stiffness. Fatigue may become more noticeable than pain. These shifts can feel like new issues, even when they reflect the body reorganizing how it copes with load and demand.

Context plays a larger role now. Poor sleep, emotional strain, or mentally heavy days can amplify physical signals without indicating a setback. At this stage, concern usually means you are paying attention, not that something is wrong. Learning to notice patterns without assigning meaning to every sensation helps interpretation stay calmer.

Patterns That Feel Wrong, Even When They're Common

Not everything that unsettles you at this stage signals trouble. Some of the most concerning experiences are patterns rather than single symptoms, and they feel alarming because they don't follow a simple story of steady improvement.

Delayed discomfort is one of the most common examples. You move through a day feeling relatively fine, only to notice symptoms later that evening or the next morning. That delay can make it seem as if something unexpected went wrong. More often, it reflects how the body processes total load over time rather than reacting immediately.

Inconsistency is another frequent source of doubt. An activity that felt manageable yesterday feels irritating today, with no clear explanation. Once progress has begun, this variability can feel like backsliding. In most cases, it points to a system that is still sensitive to cumulative demand, sleep quality, and background stress.

Fluctuating swelling fits into this pattern as well. Seeing it increase after a day that otherwise felt successful can be discouraging. At this point, swelling tends to respond more to overall volume and repetition than to any single movement, which is why cause and effect can feel disconnected.

Some patterns involve substitution rather than resolution. Pain may ease while stiffness increases. Soreness may fade as fatigue becomes more prominent. These shifts can feel like trading one problem for another, but they often reflect redistribution rather than decline.

What makes these patterns difficult is their unevenness. They are delayed, inconsistent, and sometimes contradictory. Recognizing them as common helps keep attention on overall direction rather than day-to-day noise.

When Change Matters More Than Discomfort

By this point, most people are less troubled by the fact that symptoms exist and more by how they behave. What tends to matter is not discomfort on its own, but how it changes over time.

Fluctuation usually carries less weight than persistence. Symptoms that rise and fall, even when uncomfortable, often reflect ongoing adaptation. In contrast, sensations that steadily worsen over several days or feel progressively more limiting stand out because they suggest something is not settling as expected.

A change in character can be meaningful as well. Pain that becomes sharper, more focused, or clearly different from your established pattern deserves more attention than pain that simply feels stronger on a given day. The same applies when discomfort begins to interfere with sleep in a new and persistent way.

Wider changes matter too. Feeling generally unwell, noticing warmth or redness that spreads rather than staying localized, or sensing that energy drops without rebounding can signal broader strain. These experiences are uncommon, but they tend to be clearer and more consistent than everyday soreness.

The gray area between normal fluctuation and true concern is often where anxiety grows. Seeking clarification in that space is not overreacting. Most changes that deserve attention make themselves known through persistence and pattern, not through a single bad day.

Why Direction Tells You More Than Intensity

Strong sensations naturally grab attention, but in medium-term recovery, direction usually carries more meaning than how intense something feels in the moment.

A symptom that flares and then settles often says less than one that quietly builds. Even sharp discomfort can fall within a normal range if it resolves with recovery time. When symptoms gradually worsen over several days, even without becoming severe, they suggest a trend rather than a reaction.

Delayed responses fit this pattern as well. Feeling worse a day after activity can seem confusing, especially when nothing felt wrong at the time. This lag often reflects accumulated load rather than a single misstep, which is why judging progress by one moment can be misleading.

Repetition adds another layer. A sensation that appears once and fades usually carries little weight. One that returns in the same pattern begins to carry information. Over time, these repetitions sketch direction, even when individual days feel uneven.

Focusing on direction shifts attention away from tracking every spike and toward watching how things settle overall. When symptoms fluctuate but return to baseline, recovery is usually moving forward, even if it does not feel smooth.

Rebuilding Trust in How Your Body Signals

After weeks of close monitoring, confidence in reading your own body often thins out. Not trust in the surgery itself, but trust in your ability to interpret what you feel without assuming the worst. When symptoms have been inconsistent, that confidence is easy to lose.

Earlier on, vigilance was protective. Everything was unfamiliar, and caution helped you get through. Now, the same level of monitoring can become draining. You may notice yourself scanning for problems, replaying recent days, or second-guessing sensations that once felt straightforward.

Trust returns through recognition, not reassurance. Over time, patterns become familiar. You start to recognize what a typical sore day feels like, how fatigue behaves when it is expected, and how your body usually settles after a flare. Each cycle of rise and resolution adds quiet evidence that wobble does not equal collapse.

It can help to notice what has become more reliable. Recovery time may be shorter than it used to be. Symptoms may follow a more predictable rhythm. Discomfort may feel irritating rather than alarming. These shifts often appear before confidence returns consciously.

Relearning how to trust your signals is gradual. It rarely feels like a clear decision. More often, it shows up as mental space returning, as the urge to interpret every sensation slowly loosens.

Orientation Before the Next Phase

By now, recovery usually feels less mysterious, even if it is not fully comfortable. You have lived with enough variation to recognize that symptoms rise and fall. You have seen patterns repeat. What once felt alarming now carries more context.

This chapter is not meant to turn you into an evaluator of every sensation. It offers a way of thinking. Most experiences at this stage reflect adaptation. A smaller number deserve attention. The difference usually lies in persistence, repetition, and change over time, not in how strong something feels on a single day.

Confidence often settles last. Not confidence that everything will be perfect, but confidence that you can read what is happening without panic. That steadiness grows as your body continues to respond, recover, and stabilize again and again.

Recovery does not become silent as you move forward. Signals remain part of the process. What changes is how much weight they carry. Ordinary sensations lose urgency. The few that matter tend to stand out more clearly against the background.

As you move on from here, certainty is not the goal. Orientation is. Knowing roughly where you are, what usually passes, and when clarity helps is enough to reduce the mental load recovery has carried for so long.

PART FOUR

RETURNING TO DAILY LIFE

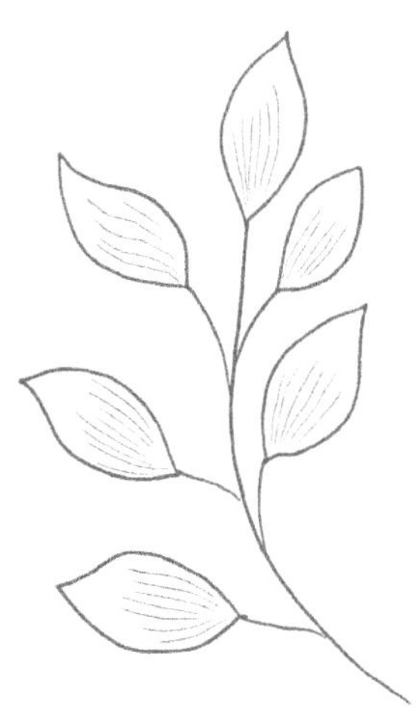

15

Walking, Stairs, Driving, and Sleep

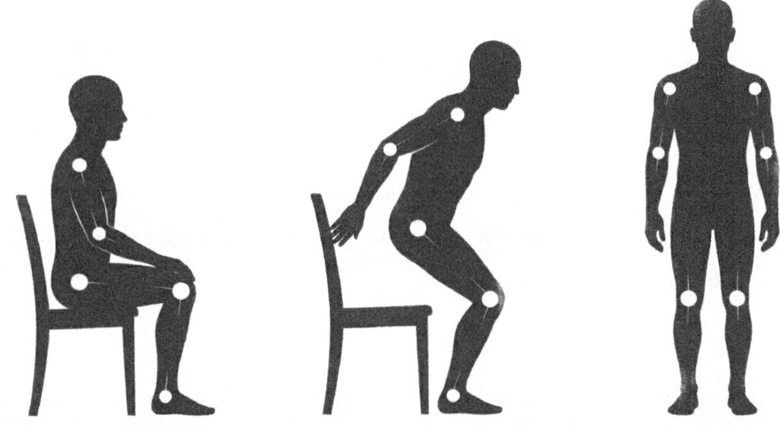

Walking seems basic. You've done it your whole life, and the joint itself may already feel capable. What often gets missed is that walking is not just strength or range of motion. It's coordination, timing, and constant prediction—your body adjusting to small changes with every step.

After surgery, those systems are still recalibrating. The joint may tolerate the load, but the nervous system works harder to manage balance and rhythm. That effort doesn't always register as pain. It often shows up as fatigue, stiffness later in the day, or a walk that feels heavier than expected.

This is why walking can feel uneven. One day it's smooth and unremarkable. The next, it feels guarded again. Strength doesn't disappear overnight, but coordination and trust fluctuate as the system decides how much attention the task still requires.

The cost of walking also tends to appear later. During the walk, things may feel fine. Hours afterward, the effort becomes noticeable. That delay can make it tempting to blame the walk itself, when what you're feeling is energy spent quietly in the background.

Walking usually becomes easier when it stops being evaluated. When it's no longer used as proof that things are going well—or not. The effort you notice is not failure. It's the price of turning an automatic skill back into a background one.

Stairs: Strength Is There, Timing Is Still Catching Up

Stairs often feel out of proportion to everything else. You may be walking comfortably and still hesitate when you reach a flight of steps. That mismatch is common.

What makes stairs demanding isn't just load. It's asymmetry and timing. One leg commits while the other stabilizes, and the movement continues without many chances to pause. Going down adds another layer, asking the body to control speed while accepting weight.

Even when the joint is physically capable, the nervous system tends to stay more alert during stairs. That extra vigilance can show up as hesitation, slower pace, or a stronger reliance on the handrail.

Context matters more than people expect. Familiar stairs at home often feel manageable, while public staircases with different heights, lighting, or people nearby can bring caution back. That difference reflects coordination and attention, not weakness.

Because stairs look effortful from the outside, they're easy to judge harshly. Using a railing or moving carefully can feel like falling behind. In reality, those choices simply reduce load while timing and trust continue to settle.

Stairs are often one of the last everyday movements to feel ordinary again. When they still require thought, it doesn't mean walking has stalled. It usually means confidence is still catching up to ability.

Driving: When Ability Returns Before Ease

Driving restores independence all at once. That's why it can feel heavier than expected, even when getting into the car, steering, or using the pedals feels manageable.

The physical actions of driving are rarely the main issue. What takes more energy is sustained attention. Driving requires constant scanning, quick decisions, and readiness to respond. After surgery, the nervous system is already working with less reserve, so that added responsibility raises the cost.

Short, familiar drives often feel easier than longer or busier ones. This isn't avoidance. It's the system easing back into a task that doesn't allow for partial effort. A tense drive doesn't mean you weren't ready—it reflects how alert the system still is.

Confidence tends to build quietly here. One trip passes without incident. Then another. Not because something was proven, but because nothing demanded proof.

Fatigue related to driving often shows up later, after the task is done. When that happens, it can be confusing, but it fits with how mental and physical load combine during recovery.

Driving usually settles when attention fades from the movement itself. Until then, caution isn't a setback. It's how independence returns without being rushed.

Sleep: Rest That Isn't Fully Restorative Yet

Sleep is expected to restore energy, yet during recovery it can still feel effortful. Even when nights are better than before, they may leave you feeling less refreshed than you'd expect.

After surgery, sleep is often fragmented. The body changes position more carefully, and the nervous system stays more alert. These brief disruptions aren't always remembered in the morning, but they reduce the depth of rest.

As daytime activity increases, sleep can become unpredictable. Doing more can support better rest overall, while also bringing temporary nighttime restlessness. That response doesn't mean you misjudged your limits. It reflects a system still adjusting how it balances activity and recovery.

Fatigue linked to sleep often shows up later in the day. Mornings may feel manageable, while energy fades faster in the afternoon or evening.

Sleep tends to improve in pieces—longer stretches, fewer sharp awakenings, less effort to reposition. What usually comes last is consistency. Nights even out gradually, without a clear moment when sleep feels "normal" again.

Why Everyday Life Still Feels Expensive

As walking, stairs, driving, and sleep return, it's easy to turn them into silent tests. When one of them feels harder than expected, it can seem as if recovery has stalled. In reality, these activities draw from the same limited energy budget.

After surgery, the body spends more effort on coordination, monitoring, and adjustment than it used to. Tasks that once ran automatically now require background attention. That added load often appears later as fatigue, heaviness, or the sense that the day took more out of you than it should have.

This is also why days vary. Energy isn't fully reset each morning. Sleep quality, stress, and the accumulation of small demands all affect how much reserve you have. A harder day doesn't erase progress from an easier one. It reflects a system still balancing supply and demand.

Using single activities as benchmarks adds pressure without clarity. Being able to do something once doesn't mean it will feel the same every day. In recovery, consistency over time matters more than performance in the moment.

As daily life becomes less supervised, effort gradually drops. Not because you push through, but because tasks stop requiring active management. When ordinary things start to feel ordinary again, it's usually because the cost has gone down—not because you passed a test.

16

Work, Social Life, and Other People's Expectations

You can sit, stand, walk, and get through tasks that once felt out of reach. On paper, that looks like readiness. What often feels uncertain instead is how long that capacity will last once the day fills up.

Work and daily routines ask for sustained effort, not short bursts. There are fewer pauses, fewer chances to reset without explanation. Attention is split, decisions stack up, and the day no longer bends around recovery. Even familiar tasks can feel heavier when they have to be carried without interruption.

This is where many people notice the gap between being able to do something and being able to do it repeatedly. The joint may tolerate the movement, but endurance for full days is still catching up. Questions about how the body will feel later tend to run quietly in the background, adding strain without being obvious.

Mental effort draws from the same reserve as physical healing. Concentration, problem-solving, and staying socially engaged all cost energy. When those demands return before stamina is fully rebuilt, fatigue shows up sooner—not as pain, but as a sense of being spent.

That unevenness is common. It usually settles through ordinary exposure rather than pressure. As days pass without consequences, confidence follows. Feeling mentally heavier than expected at this point is rarely a sign of weakness. It reflects endurance rebuilding under real conditions, which takes longer than regaining basic ability.

Why Interaction Costs More Than Movement

A short conversation can leave you more tired than a walk. That contrast often feels confusing, especially when pain is no longer the main issue.

Social situations demand steady attention. You're listening, responding, tracking cues, adjusting posture, and staying present all at once. Unlike physical tasks, there's less room to change position, step away, or slow the pace without it being noticed. Even pleasant interactions ask for sustained focus.

Many people become more aware of their body around others than they are at home. Where to sit. How long to stand. Whether shifting looks awkward. That quiet self-checking runs continuously in the background, using energy even when nothing goes wrong.

Kind comments can add another layer. Being told you look great or seem "back to normal" can create pressure to match that picture. Enjoyment and monitoring start competing for space. The effort isn't emotional weakness; it's attention being stretched thin.

Earlier, reduced social contact made sense and was clearly justified. As participation increases, comfort doesn't always keep the same pace. Tolerance for layered demands is still rebuilding. When interaction feels draining before it feels natural, that's a common bridge phase—not a change in personality or resilience.

When Being "Almost Fine" Raises the Bar

Showing up again sends a strong signal. At work or in social settings, presence often gets read as proof that recovery is complete. From the outside, that conclusion makes sense. You're moving better. You're participating. You look steady.

Inside, things still feel conditional. Energy varies. Confidence depends on context. What you can do once doesn't always translate into what you can repeat day after day. When others assume consistency before it's there, pressure shifts from getting through the task to performing stability.

That pressure matters because the body responds to it. Monitoring yourself more closely, anticipating how you'll feel later, or trying to avoid visible strain all increase nervous system alertness. When that system stays on guard, symptoms like fatigue, stiffness, or vague discomfort can rise even without extra physical load.

Support also changes quietly at this point. Earlier, adjustments were expected. Now they're less visible, even though they still help. Hesitation can start to feel like something that needs justification, which adds another layer of effort.

This mirrors patterns you've already seen with movement. Confidence builds through ordinary experiences that don't cost you afterward, not through meeting an outside picture of being "done." When expectations arrive before internal readiness, the strain you feel is real and physical, not a failure to cope.

How Pressure Shows Up in the Body

You can handle the activity, yet feel worse later. That delay often makes it hard to connect cause and effect.

External pressure—being observed, evaluated, or relied on—keeps attention turned outward while the body is still adjusting. The system stays slightly braced, tracking performance and outcome rather than settling into the task itself. That constant alert state uses energy, even when movement stays within safe limits.

Stress doesn't need to feel dramatic to have an effect. Mild tension, held for hours, can amplify fatigue and physical sensations. The body reads expectation as demand, and demand as something to prepare for. Over time, that preparation shows up as stiffness, heaviness, or exhaustion.

This is why symptoms can appear on days that look reasonable on the surface. Nothing was "too much" in isolation. It was the combination of activity, attention, and pressure layered together. When that stack exceeds current tolerance, the response is physiological, not personal.

As tolerance grows, this pattern softens. The nervous system learns that full participation doesn't require constant vigilance. When symptoms start arriving later, or fading faster, it usually signals that this learning is underway—even if the days still feel uneven.

The Quiet Cost of Holding It Together

By the time days start to look normal again, effort becomes less visible. You're working, talking, moving through full schedules. From the outside, there's little to point to as demanding.

What often goes unnoticed is the work of maintaining that appearance. Staying attentive, keeping pace, managing posture and movement without obvious adjustment—all of that runs quietly in the background. It doesn't announce itself as strain, but it still draws from the same reserve that recovery depends on.

This is why fatigue at this stage can feel out of proportion. It arrives later, sometimes the next day, and lingers without a clear trigger. It isn't the exhaustion of early healing. It's the accumulation of layered demands returning faster than endurance can absorb them.

People often read this as a setback. In most cases, it isn't. Ability tends to return before stamina. The gap shows up as tiredness rather than pain, especially when full participation resumes.

As days repeat without consequence, the cost gradually drops. Attention loosens. Monitoring fades. Fatigue arrives later and resolves sooner. When that happens, it may not feel like progress—but it's one of the clearest signs that recovery is settling into daily life.

17

Trusting Your New Joint

The joint is moving. Daily tasks are mostly back in place. Pain no longer sets the tone of the day. And yet hesitation still shows up. That pause can be hard to explain, especially when there's no clear reason for it.

This gap between what the joint can do and how safe it feels is one of the most common features of late recovery. Function often improves first. Trust tends to follow later. When the two don't line up, it's easy to assume something is unfinished.

What's happening is not doubt about strength or stability. It's a lag in expectation. For a long time, movement required caution. The body learned to anticipate problems before sensation appeared. Even when the joint no longer needs that protection, the expectation doesn't reset on command.

This is why reassurance rarely closes the gap. Being told the joint is "fine" doesn't remove the pause. Trust doesn't respond to explanation. It adjusts through repeated experiences that end without consequence.

Confidence usually becomes visible only in hindsight. You realize later that you moved without planning, without bracing, without slowing yourself down. Those moments don't stand out when they happen. They quietly accumulate in the background.

When confidence is expected to lead, pressure builds. In practice, it almost always trails behind. Trust grows through use that no longer asks for attention.

Hesitation Without Pain Still Carries Weight

"I know it's strong, but..." is a familiar thought at this point. You start a routine movement and notice a brief beat of hesitation. There's no pain. Nothing feels unstable. Still, the body slows things down.

This kind of hesitation often feels more unsettling than pain. Pain has a clear logic. It points to something concrete. Hesitation without pain feels vague, which makes people question it or try to override it. If nothing hurts, reluctance can seem out of place.

What's lagging here isn't healing. It's anticipation. The body spent a long time learning when not to commit fully. That learning was useful when the joint was unreliable. Even now, the process that approves movement is still double-checking.

These moments tend to appear when commitment matters. A quick turn. An uneven surface. A step that can't easily be reversed once it starts. The joint may tolerate the load, but the approval arrives a fraction later than expected.

Occasional symptoms complicate this learning. A random ache later in the day. Brief stiffness after rest. A heavy feeling that fades on its own. Even mild sensations can interrupt confidence because unexpected signals carry more weight than many neutral ones.

Trying to force confidence usually makes the moment louder. When movement becomes a test, the experience stops being neutral. When the pause is allowed and the movement proceeds without pressure, the outcome matters more than the feeling beforehand.

Hesitation without pain isn't a warning. It's part of how expectations are revised. Trust returns not because reluctance disappears first, but because the hesitation stops being reinforced.

Feeling Capable, Then Suddenly Less Sure

Progress doesn't always feel like momentum. In fact, confidence often dips just as function improves. You can do more, move more freely, and rely on the joint more often—yet uncertainty becomes easier to notice.

The reason is simple: the stakes change. Earlier on, limits were obvious. Movements were slow, deliberate, and carefully managed. As capacity grows, situations become less controlled. You move faster. You react instead of planning. That shift exposes the gap between what the joint can handle and how quickly approval arrives.

Feedback changes as well. Strong pain and stiffness once provided constant information. As those signals fade, what remains is quieter and less predictable. The body is still communicating, but with less clarity. That can feel unsettling, even though it reflects improvement rather than decline.

Delayed feedback adds another layer. A movement may feel fine in the moment, then show up hours later as soreness or fatigue. When cause and effect are separated in time, learning slows. A single delayed symptom can outweigh many uneventful actions.

This is why confidence doesn't rise in a straight line. It dips, stabilizes, then dips again as new situations are added. Each dip isn't a loss of trust. It's the body being asked to update expectations under slightly different conditions.

What makes this confusing is that nothing obvious fixes it. Uneven confidence here doesn't mean progress has stalled. It means the joint is being used in a wider range of real-life contexts. The learning continues, just not all at once.

Why Trust Forms Quietly, Not on Command

You don't decide to trust a joint. You notice later that you already did.

Confidence rarely shows up as a feeling first. More often, it appears as an absence. Less monitoring before you move. Less bracing during movement. Fewer questions afterward about how it went. Nothing dramatic changes in the moment, which is why it's easy to miss.

Repetition matters more than intention. The body updates safety based on what actually happens, not on what you tell yourself. Each time a movement unfolds without needing correction, expectations shift slightly. Over time, those small shifts outweigh older habits of caution.

Because this learning is quiet, it's easily disrupted by attention. Actively checking for confidence pulls focus back to uncertainty. Monitoring every sensation turns neutral experiences into charged ones. When movement blends into the day without commentary, trust has room to settle.

Fatigue influences this process as well. When energy is lower, the body becomes more conservative. Confidence can feel reduced even though capacity hasn't changed. That swing is often mistaken for regression, when it's really a temporary narrowing of tolerance.

Trust doesn't grow evenly or permanently. It forms in layers, shaped by context, energy, and recent experience. Some situations settle sooner than others. That unevenness isn't a flaw in recovery. It's how learning works once real life replaces controlled conditions.

When the Joint Stops Being the Reference Point

The clearest sign that trust is forming is not confidence. It's distraction.

At some point, the joint stops being the main thing you check in with during the day. You still rely on it, but it no longer anchors your awareness. Attention shifts outward—toward what you're doing, who you're with, what comes next. The joint is present, but no longer central.

This doesn't mean sensations disappear. Small aches, stiffness after rest, or end-of-day fatigue can still show up. What changes is their weight. They pass without being evaluated or tied to meaning. Movement happens without rehearsal. You don't replay the day to judge how the joint behaved.

Earlier, attention served a purpose. It helped protect you while outcomes were uncertain. Now, that same level of monitoring can keep uncertainty alive. Letting the joint fade into the background isn't neglect. It's integration.

Many people worry that easing attention means missing something important. In practice, meaningful problems tend to make themselves known. What fades instead is the background noise—the checking, the bracing, the quiet second-guessing.

Trust doesn't arrive as certainty or completion. It settles as normalcy. The joint becomes part of the body again, not the measure of every decision. Recovery, at this point, isn't finished—but it is workable. And that steadiness is enough to carry things forward without needing to keep score.

PART FOUR

LOOKING AHEAD

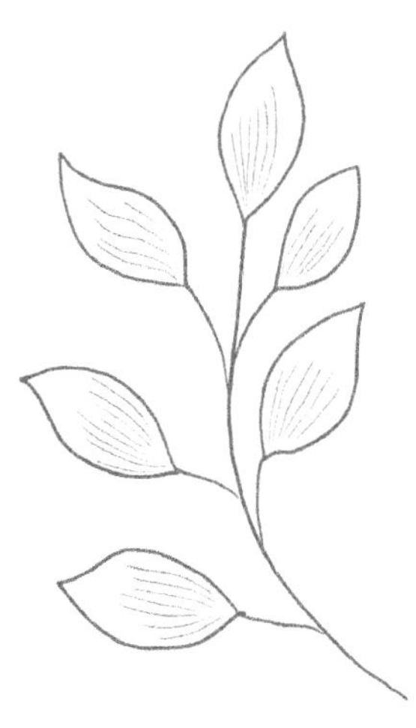

18

Long-Term Recovery and Joint Care

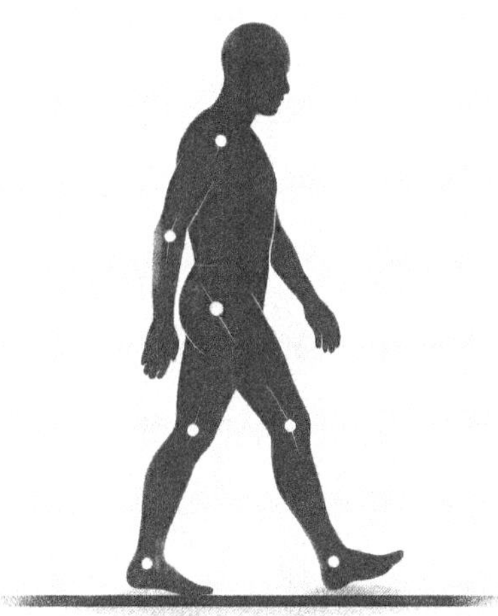

There is a point when the joint no longer organizes your thinking. Not because it feels perfect, and not because sensations have vanished, but because it no longer demands constant decisions. You move through the day without checking first, and only notice afterward that you didn't think about it at all.

Earlier on, attention had a purpose. Monitoring pain, swelling, and fatigue helped you navigate uncertainty. Over time, that same focus can outlive its usefulness. When vigilance stays in place longer than needed, recovery can feel unfinished even when the body has already adapted.

Most people recognize this shift indirectly. An errand done without planning. A change of direction without bracing. Standing up quickly and realizing there was no pause. These moments rarely feel important. They're easy to overlook. But they mark a real change in how the joint fits into daily life.

Letting go of constant checking can feel unfamiliar after months of close attention. Some worry that less awareness means being careless. It doesn't. The body is no longer asking for the same level of supervision because it no longer relies on it.

Sensations may still appear. Mild stiffness, a brief ache, a reminder at the end of a long day. The difference is not their absence, but their weight. They pass without analysis. They don't interrupt the day or ask for interpretation.

Living this way doesn't mean ignoring your body. It means trusting that it will signal clearly when something truly needs attention. Most of the time, it doesn't. And that quiet often signals that recovery has shifted into a different phase.

What "Normal" Gradually Becomes

Later on, normal is often less dramatic than expected. Most people feel more capable than they did before surgery. Movement flows more easily. Daily tasks cost less effort. At the same time, the joint may still make itself known occasionally—not as a problem, but as part of the background.

This can be surprising. Many assume that enough time should erase all sensation. When it doesn't, it's easy to wonder whether something stalled. In reality, long-term recovery tends to settle rather than conclude.

Variation becomes part of that settled state. Some days are almost forgettable. Others include stiffness, heaviness, or fatigue without a clear trigger. These shifts are usually brief. They don't point to decline. They reflect a body that is active, responsive, and still adjusting to changing demands.

What matters most is not how the joint feels in a single moment, but how it behaves across time. Discomfort resolves more quickly. Rest restores function. Activity no longer sets off a chain reaction. Those patterns carry more meaning than isolated sensations.

This is often when the question changes. Instead of "Is this okay?" it becomes "This passes." That shift reduces background noise. It allows response without commentary and movement without negotiation.

Normal, at this stage, isn't a fixed endpoint. It's stability. An understanding that fluctuation is part of living in a body, not a sign that something is wrong. Once that expectation settles, the joint takes up far less space in your thinking.

When Activity Returns to the Background

Movement works differently once recovery has blended back into daily life. It no longer needs tracking, counting, or evaluation. Walking, standing, lifting, changing direction—these return to being part of the day rather than something set apart and observed.

Earlier on, measuring made sense. Progress felt uncertain, and numbers offered reassurance. Over time, that same focus can keep attention fixed on the joint, even when it no longer needs it. The body already regulates effort well when it isn't being watched so closely.

Many people notice a quiet urge to keep score. Steps taken. Time spent. Whether today was "enough." This mindset often lingers out of habit rather than need. When it stays in place, it adds pressure without improving comfort or function.

Long-term steadiness comes from responsiveness, not control. Activity naturally rises and falls with the day, the week, and life itself. Adjusting without explanation is one of the clearest signs that recovery has integrated into everyday living.

Staying active doesn't mean staying busy. It means staying connected to what fits your life again. Activities that feel natural tend to continue. Those that feel imposed tend to fade, regardless of how carefully they're planned.

When movement stops being something you evaluate, it becomes something you trust. That trust doesn't announce itself. It simply allows the day to unfold without the joint needing to stay in focus.

Care Without Guarding

Long-term care often turns out to be simpler than expected. By this point, the joint has shown you how it responds. You recognize what feels ordinary and what feels different. That familiarity replaces rules, and care becomes situational rather than constant.

Guarding can resemble caution, but it carries a different tone. Movements stay tentative. The joint is treated as fragile, even after it has demonstrated reliability. Over time, that stance can limit confidence more than the joint itself ever would.

Care works differently. If the joint feels tired, you ease off without concern. If it feels stiff, you move and it settles. If something lingers, you notice it without immediately assigning meaning. Most of the time, no further response is required.

This reflects how long-term adaptation unfolds. Tissues continue adjusting to load through ordinary use, gradually becoming more tolerant. Sensitivity may fluctuate at times, but that reflects responsiveness rather than damage.

As unnecessary caution fades, many people notice a shift in tone. The joint is no longer something to defend. It's something you live with. It doesn't need constant reassurance, and it doesn't ask for it.

When care replaces guarding, confidence grows without effort—not because you are doing more, but because you are allowing the body to do what it already knows how to do.

A Quieter Kind of Confidence

Confidence, at this stage, rarely feels dramatic. It doesn't arrive as certainty or boldness. It shows up as ease. As fewer pauses. As less internal commentary during ordinary movement.

You act without checking first. You adjust without labeling it. You trust that if something truly needs attention, it will become clear. Most of the time, it doesn't. That absence is meaningful.

This kind of confidence isn't built by testing limits or proving anything. It forms when daily life proceeds smoothly enough that the joint no longer needs a voice in every decision. You don't think about trusting it. You simply move, and nothing pushes back.

There may still be moments of awareness. A long day. An unfamiliar surface. A movement that feels slightly different than expected. These moments register, then pass. They don't change how safe you feel in your body.

Over time, the joint becomes ordinary. Not invisible, but unremarkable. It functions. It adapts. It supports what you want to do without requiring supervision.

For many people, this is what long-term recovery actually looks like: not a finish line, and not a return to before, but a stable, workable relationship with the body.

When the Story Quietly Closes

Eventually, there is no longer an active recovery to manage. The joint works as part of you now. It has a role, but it no longer shapes your decisions or frames your day.

Recovery doesn't announce its ending. Most people don't notice a clear moment of arrival. They recognize it later, by absence—by how little space the joint occupies, by how rarely it enters their thoughts, by how ordinary movement has become.

Daily life continues with its usual variation. Some days are lighter. Others are more demanding. The joint responds as part of that rhythm, not as something separate that requires watching.

A good long-term outcome isn't vigilance or effort. It isn't progress you have to defend. It's stability that holds on its own, without constant attention.

That kind of stability simply supports the life around it.
And that is enough.

19

Redefining a Successful Recovery

At some point, the idea of getting back loses its hold. Early on, it can feel like the only way to judge whether recovery has worked at all. A familiar version of yourself becomes the reference point. Over time, that comparison starts to strain. Not because the past no longer matters, but because it no longer matches the body you're living in now.

The body has changed in quiet ways. Not just the joint itself, but how effort accumulates, how rest restores, how movement settles afterward. Measuring success against an earlier version can keep dissatisfaction active even when daily life is functioning well.

Many people notice a shift when the question changes. Less about whether something feels the same as before, and more about whether it works. Can you move through the day without managing symptoms? Can you make plans without bracing for them? Can you expect tomorrow to resemble today closely enough to trust it?

Letting go of "back to before" is not lowering the bar. It's adjusting the frame. It allows stability to count as progress, and predictability to matter more than perfect comfort. When that shift settles, success is no longer a comparison. It becomes a condition that remains steady.

What Holds, Day After Day

Long-term success rarely announces itself. It doesn't arrive with a clear signal or a moment worth marking. It shows up indirectly, through days that no longer demand attention.

Routines begin to run without adjustment. You move through mornings, errands, and evenings without structuring them around the joint. When discomfort appears, it fits within a familiar range and resolves without changing how you approach the next day.

Pain-free is not the standard here. Fluctuation still exists. A stiff start that loosens. A heavier afternoon that fades by evening. What changes is not the presence of sensation, but its weight. These variations stop carrying meaning. They no longer suggest decline or require interpretation.

Reliability becomes the quiet measure. Knowing how your body responds. Knowing that effort does not spiral. Knowing that rest restores rather than resets everything. This predictability allows attention to move elsewhere.

Ease emerges without effort, often noticed only in hindsight. Not ease as lightness, but ease as lack of friction. Movement without negotiation. Activity without recovery accounting afterward. When daily life runs without commentary, success is already in place.

Independence Without Demonstration

Independence, by this stage, has very little to prove. It no longer depends on showing what you can do or confirming that recovery was worthwhile. It shows up as choice made without rehearsal.

Many people notice a subtle pressure linger longer than expected—the sense that ability needs to be validated. Walking farther. Staying active longer.

Saying yes to avoid doubt. As recovery settles, that pressure fades. You do what the day requires, and the joint no longer enters the calculation first.

Independence looks quieter than expected. It looks like agreeing to plans without scanning ahead for limits. Like declining without explanation. Like changing direction without feeling behind.

Nothing needs defending. Nothing needs evidence. You know what you can manage because you live it. Adjustments happen when they make sense, not because they are required. That balance doesn't rely on discipline or vigilance. It remains stable on its own.

When independence stops being something you earn, it becomes something that simply exists.

Confidence That No Longer Needs Attention

Confidence takes on a different shape here. It isn't built from reassurance, and it isn't unsettled by small changes. It doesn't ask to be checked or reinforced. It's present in how little space it occupies.

You trust your body without running through reasons. When something feels off, you respond without urgency. When it doesn't, you move on without remark. Capability and confidence have not aligned all at once, but they have gradually realigned through experience that ends without consequence.

This is the nervous system learning through consistency rather than instruction. Days that resolve themselves. Patterns that remain dependable without supervision. The joint no longer requires constant awareness, and that absence is not neglect. It's a sign that monitoring is no longer needed to stay safe.

Confidence here is not a feeling to protect. It's a background state that allows life to proceed uninterrupted. Minor sensations may still appear, but they don't organize your thinking. Ongoing awareness does not mean recovery has failed. It means the body is still adapting while life continues to move forward.

When the Story Closes Quietly

Recovery does not end with a final test or a moment worth marking. It fades from the center of attention on its own. The joint finds its place in your life, and life fills in around it.

Movement, comfort, and ability continue to exist, but they no longer organize your day. They function in the background, adjusting as needed, without demanding supervision. There is no standard to maintain and no outcome to protect. What works remains stable because it is lived, not managed.

This book does not need to stay open to remain useful. Some people return to it later, not because something has gone wrong, but because perspective shifts over time. Reading again can clarify orientation rather than reopen questions.

What remains is ordinary life, resumed without commentary. Days that move forward without checking back. The story closes not because everything is finished, but because it no longer needs telling.

Appendix – Recovery Glossary

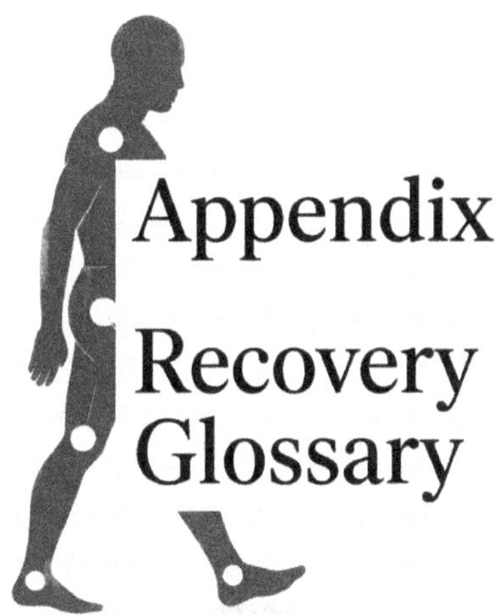

The terms in this glossary appear throughout the guide, in conversations with physical therapists, or in your own thinking during recovery. They are included here to clarify meaning, not to add rules or expectations.

You do not need to read this section from beginning to end. It is meant to be used selectively, when a word stands out or feels unclear. The definitions focus on lived experience rather than technical detail.

Language shapes how recovery is understood. Having words for common sensations, patterns, and responses can make the process easier to recognize without overanalyzing it. This glossary is here to support orientation, not monitoring.

———◆○◆———

Adaptation

The body's ability to adjust over time to new demands, positions, or loads. In recovery, adaptation often shows up as gradual tolerance rather than immediate comfort. Changes may be subtle and uneven, but they reflect learning rather than strain.

Awareness

The degree of attention you give to the joint during movement or daily activities. Increased awareness is common after surgery and does not mean something is wrong. Over time, awareness usually fades as movement becomes more automatic.

Baseline

Your usual level of comfort, ability, and energy on an average day. The baseline is not a perfect day, but a familiar one. Recovery often shows up as a more stable baseline rather than constant improvement.

Capacity

What the body can handle at a given time, physically and mentally. Capacity includes strength, endurance, and recovery ability. It can improve before it becomes consistent.

Compensation

A change in how you move to protect a joint or reduce discomfort. Compensation is often temporary and adaptive early on. It becomes less noticeable as confidence and movement efficiency return.

Confidence

Trust in your body's ability to move without causing harm. Confidence usually lags behind physical improvement and builds through repeated, uneventful experiences. It tends to show up as reduced hesitation rather than increased boldness.

Consistency

How reliably your body responds from day to day. Consistency matters more than peak performance in long-term recovery. Small fluctuations can exist without undermining overall stability.

Discomfort

Unpleasant sensations that fall short of pain, such as soreness, tightness, or pressure. Discomfort is common during adaptation and does not automatically signal injury. Its significance depends more on pattern than intensity.

Endurance

The ability to sustain activity over time without excessive fatigue or symptom flare. Endurance often returns more slowly than strength. It usually improves through repeated exposure rather than effort alone.

Effort

The physical and mental energy required to complete an activity. After surgery, tasks may require more effort even when they are technically possible. As recovery progresses, effort decreases before movement feels fully normal.

Fatigue

A sense of tiredness or reduced capacity that is not always relieved by rest. After surgery, fatigue can reflect healing demands and nervous system effort, not just physical exertion. It often improves gradually as routines become easier.

Flare

A temporary increase in symptoms following activity, stress, or accumulated load. A flare does not necessarily indicate injury or setback. It usually settles as the body recovers and recalibrates.

Function

What you are able to do in daily life, regardless of how movement feels moment to moment. Function can improve even when some discomfort remains. In recovery, function often stabilizes before sensations fully quiet down.

Gait

The pattern of how you walk, including rhythm, balance, and coordination. Changes in gait are common after joint surgery and often reflect caution rather than weakness. As confidence returns, gait usually becomes more automatic.

Guarding

A protective response where movement becomes stiff or limited to avoid discomfort. Guarding is often unconscious and can persist after tissues have healed. It tends to ease as trust in movement rebuilds.

Healing

The ongoing process by which tissues repair and adapt after surgery. Healing does not progress at a steady pace and may continue long after symptoms change. Feeling better and being healed are related but not identical.

Inflammation

A normal response to surgery and activity that helps initiate repair. Inflammation can cause warmth, swelling, and sensitivity without signaling damage. Its presence alone does not indicate a problem.

Load

The physical demand placed on the joint through movement, posture, or

, or repetition. Load is not harmful by default. Problems arise when load exceeds what the body can comfortably recover from.

Mobility

The ability of a joint to move through its available range with ease. Mobility can be limited by stiffness, swelling, or guarding rather than structural restriction. It often improves as movement becomes less effortful.

Monitoring

The habit of frequently checking sensations, movement, or symptoms. Monitoring is common early in recovery and often fades as predictability improves. Ongoing awareness does not mean recovery has failed.

Movement Quality

How smoothly and efficiently a movement is performed. After surgery, movement quality may feel awkward or deliberate even when strength is sufficient. It often improves gradually as coordination and confidence return.

Muscle Inhibition

A temporary reduction in how effectively a muscle activates after surgery or swelling. This response is protective rather than harmful. It usually resolves as the joint tolerates movement more comfortably.

Pain

An unpleasant sensory experience that can vary in intensity, timing, and meaning during recovery. Pain does not always reflect damage or delayed healing. Its pattern over time is often more informative than its presence alone.

Pattern

The way symptoms or responses tend to repeat over time. Patterns help distinguish between temporary fluctuation and meaningful change. Recognizing patterns can reduce unnecessary concern about isolated sensations.

Predictability

The ability to anticipate how your body is likely to respond to activity or rest. Predictability matters more than perfect comfort in long-term recovery. It allows planning without constant adjustment.

Progress

Change over time that improves function, tolerance, or stability. Progress is often uneven and easier to recognize in hindsight. Short-term setbacks do not cancel longer-term gains.

Range of Motion

The amount a joint can move in different directions. Range of motion may improve before it feels natural or comfortable. Small limitations do not always interfere with daily function.

Recalibration

The process by which the body and nervous system adjust expectations after surgery. Recalibration involves learning what movements are safe again. It happens through experience rather than conscious control.

Recovery

The broader process of returning to daily life after surgery, including physical, mental, and emotional adjustment. Recovery does not follow a straight line. It often continues even after symptoms become less noticeable.

Reliability

How consistently your body responds to similar activities. Reliability allows trust to develop without constant monitoring. Minor variation can exist without undermining overall stability.

Reserve

The extra capacity the body has beyond what is needed for basic tasks. Reserve allows you to handle unexpected demands without symptoms escalating. Early in recovery, reserve is limited and gradually rebuilds.

Setback

A period when symptoms temporarily increase or function feels reduced. Setbacks are common and often reflect accumulated load rather than damage. They usually resolve as balance is restored.

Stability

The ability to move and bear weight without excessive effort or uncertainty. Stability is not about stiffness or rigidity. It reflects coordination and confidence working together.

Stiffness

A feeling of resistance when starting to move, especially after rest. Stiffness often relates to reduced circulation or guarding rather than injury. It typically eases once movement resumes.

Strength

The ability of muscles to produce force. Strength often returns earlier than endurance or confidence. Feeling strong does not always mean the system is ready for sustained activity.

Swelling

An increase in fluid around the joint following surgery or activity. Swelling can fluctuate day to day and does not always correlate with pain. Its presence alone does not indicate a problem.

Tolerance

How well the body accepts activity without prolonged symptoms. Tolerance builds gradually through repeated exposure. It is shaped by recovery ability, not just effort.

Trust

Confidence that movement can occur without harm. Trust develops through repeated experiences that end without consequence. It often lags behind physical healing.

Variability

Normal day-to-day changes in comfort, energy, or movement. Variability is expected during recovery and does not mean progress is lost. Stability can exist alongside variability.

Vigilance

A heightened state of attention toward bodily sensations or movement. Vigilance is common after surgery and reflects protection rather than weakness. It usually decreases as predictability improves.

Weight-Bearing

The act of placing body weight through the joint during standing or movement. Weight-bearing often feels demanding before it feels natural. Confidence in weight-bearing tends to return gradually.

Workload

The combined physical and mental demands placed on the body over time. Workload includes activity, posture, and daily responsibilities. Managing workload helps prevent unnecessary flare-ups.

Notes for Caregivers

If you're reading this as a caregiver, you're often the one noticing changes first. You see patterns the patient may dismiss or minimize, especially on tired or discouraged days.

Small fluctuations are common and don't always need to be fixed or explained. What helps most is staying steady—listening, observing, and avoiding quick conclusions when things feel inconsistent.

Pay attention to shifts in function and mood, not just symptoms. Increased withdrawal, growing hesitation, or trouble with everyday tasks can matter as much as physical signs.

When concerns come up, sharing what you've observed over time is often more useful than focusing on a single moment. Your calm perspective can help reduce worry rather than add to it.

Thanks

Thank you for spending time with this book.

If you're holding it at the end, it means you've likely been through something demanding—physically, mentally, or both. My goal was to offer clarity, reassurance, and a steady reference during a period that often feels uncertain and lonely.

If this guide helped you feel more oriented, less worried, or simply less alone at any point in your recovery, I would truly appreciate it if you took a moment to leave a brief review on Amazon.

Reviews help in two important ways. They support my work, allowing me to continue creating resources like this one. And they help other patients and caregivers decide whether this book might be useful for them as well—especially when they're facing similar questions or concerns.

Even a few lines are enough. Thank you for taking the time, and I wish you continued progress and steadier days ahead.

www.ingramcontent.com/pod-product-compliance
Lightning Source LLC
Chambersburg PA
CBHW051509050726
47594CB00010B/4028